Garlic
Nature's Original Remedy

Garlic

Nature's Original Remedy

Stephen Fulder
John Blackwood

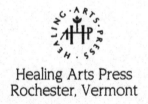

Healing Arts Press
Rochester, Vermont

Healing Arts Press
One Park Street
Rochester, Vermont
www.InnerTraditions.com

Healing Arts Press is a division of Inner Traditions International

Note to the reader: This book is intended as an informational guide. The remedies,
approaches, and techniques described herein are meant to supplement, and not
to be a substitute for, professional medical care or treatment. They should not
be used to treat a serious ailment without prior consultation with a qualified
healthcare professional.

LIBRARY OF CONGRESS CATALOGING-IN-PUBLICATION DATA
Fulder, Stephen.
    Garlic : nature's original remedy / Stephen Fulder, John Blackwood.
        p. cm.
    Includes bibliographical references and index.
    ISBN 978-0-89281-725-2
    1. Garlic—Therapeutic use. 2. Garlic. I. Blackwood, John. II. Title.
RM666.G15F85   1991
615'.324324—dc20   91-8673
                                                                 CIP

Printed and bound in the United States

10   9   8

Contents

Acknowledgments

The authors would like to thank the following people for their assistance and support: Mr. David Backhouse and Mr. David Roser of Hofels Pure Foods Ltd., Mr. Anton Graf of Madaus Murdoch Inc., Vicomtesse Anoushka d'Amonville, Mr. Dick Barker, Professor William Blackwood, Dr. D. J. Boullin, Monsignor David Greenstock, Dr. Anthony Hyder, Dr. A. Nibbi, Mr. Arthur Oaks, Lama Chime Radha, Dr. Lance Cousins, Dr. Malcolm Stuart, Mr. Richard Temple and the library staff of the Royal Horticultural Society, London, and the Department of Botany, Oxford University.

Authors' Note

This book presents the case for a place for garlic in general health care. Readers should not take suggestions concerning its use as prescriptions for specific health problems. Likewise, we are not attempting to judge and compare remedies for specific diagnosed conditions, but only to weigh general advantages and disadvantages. Those with health problems should always seek professional assistance.

1

Garlic Presented

Man's relationship with garlic is extremely ancient. Its bulb is pungent, energy-giving, and easy to store, and would have had an immediate appeal as a food. Then, by trial and error, by inspiration or by accident, man would have discovered its power to heal infections and cure disease. It may well have been one of his first remedies. Could it have been discovered in this way?

> The rain beat upon the yurt, making the felt sides hang heavily. The sound of water came from far away also, as the snows melted and streams rushed down the mountainsides. The man sat inside, with his wife and small son.
>
> Next day, the man began to shiver and his body ached. He lay helpless, wracked with pain. He became light-headed, and his soul passed from him, out through the smoke opening and away over the high ground strewn with boulders. A demoness pursued him. She had one eye and one ear and her hair was like the branches of thorn bushes. Her hair was flecked with blood.

The woman went to the *kam,* the wise man. "Call back his soul," she begged. He beat his drum and sang spirit songs so that he might enter the land of shadows. He rode the long-necked bird to the door of the Land of the Dead, to the gate of Erlik's kingdom. The demoness was wrestling with the man's soul, trying to drag him in.

Beside the gate a plant grew. Its leaves were long and sharp; its flowers were purple and its round head grew in the ground. The kam wondered at the plant but recognized its power. He pulled it up, broke off three pieces from the head and threw them into the sky. They hung there like crescent moons.

They made a loud sound in the sky, like gongs, and they distracted the demoness's attention. The kam had tricked her. He lifted the man onto the back of the bird.

To return was hard. Crossing the red desert, they grew tired. Crossing the iron mountain, they fell to earth. They were caught in a narrow place, without escape. So the kam took more pieces of the plant and fed them to the bird. Its strength revived and they flew home.

The man still lay in fever but his soul had returned to him. The kam went out to find the plant which he had seen in his vision. He brought it to the woman. "Break the pieces of the head and put them in a soup for your husband." She crushed the cloves and their smell filled the yurt. The man sweated more, but his fever left him.

Then the people of that tribe gathered the plant and later they grew it for themselves. They found it good to eat and good for many illnesses. All the tribes carried it with them on their journeyings for strength and for healing.

Could there be any truth in this tale of garlic's origins as medicinal plant? There are many legends of similar dream-inspired discoveries—of ginseng, for example, and of the coca plant. Moreover, we have tried to give it the flavor of

Central Asian shamanism because it is from that region that botanists believe garlic to have come. The area in question lies north of Afghanistan and northwest of Tibet, at the meeting of the southern borders of Russia and the western borders of China. It has always been a crossroads of humanity. Hun and Mongol conquerors swept through. Alexander the Great passed that way to India.

Amongst the many explorers of that region were the Russian botanists Alexis and Olga Fedtschenko, who discovered many specimens of plants from the botanical group to which garlic belongs, the genus *Allium*. The majority were found growing in the narrow gorges which provide access to the great mountain ranges. One, called *Allium longicuspis*, had, in almost every respect, the same appearance as the garlic we know. Here and nowhere else in the world was the garlic plant growing in an originally wild state. From here, man first gathered and grew it, and from here it spread around the world.

It may seem strange to connect garlic with the mountains of Central Asia rather than the sunny shores of the Mediterranean, but in fact it adapts extremely well to different climates and will grow in most regions of the world, except the Arctic and moist equatorial jungles. It has always been a part of life in those high regions. Caravan men chew cloves of garlic as an antidote to altitude sickness and, in Tibet, it is fermented with butter and grain to produce a general-purpose medicine. In cold weather, it strengthens the heart of the traveler. In his book *High Tartary*, Owen Lattimore gives the following description of Chang's Vinegar Shop in Ku Ch'eng-tze, Zungaria, which he visited in the winter of 1927. It is a scene which must have remained unchanged for centuries.

The daily terms included two full meals, with free shao-chiu [distilled grain spirit], camel owners and camel pullers messing in common at four-man tables in the huge kitchen, in a snug frowst of steaming men warmed by roaring ovens. From the smoke-blackened rafters, glistening like dark enamel in the gloom overhead, depended strings of garlic, and the cooks breathed equality, fraternity, and garlic as they rushed from table to table with renewed platters of garlic laden chiao-tze—steamed meat patties—and saucers of grilled sliced mutton and fried onions, dishes of sauce and vinegar, and stacks of puffy steamed rolls.

Moreover, by some coincidence of history, some quirk of fate, garlic has a double connection with the Eastern Turkistan of the late nineteenth century. In 1890, Lt. Bower, a young Indian Army officer, was traveling in that region. He was approached by a Turki who offered to sell him an ancient manuscript consisting of sheets of birch bark inscribed in Sanskrit. He had found it sealed inside a crumbling mound of brick and wood, close to an extensive series of cave dwellings hollowed out of the side of a nearby hill. When this text (now known as the Bower manuscript) was taken back to Calcutta, it caused something of a sensation. It was found to be a medical treatise copied down between AD 350 and 375, and was therefore the oldest Sanskrit manuscript in existence.

It provides a wonderful introduction to garlic lore. It begins with a description of the sacred mountain where healing plants grow.

Om! In your beautiful groves, resounding with the voices of various kinds of birds, the medicinal plants glow at night like sacrificial fires.

On that mountain which is, through its gifts, the bene-
factor of all creatures, there dwell the sages of enlightened
mind. These roam the countryside in company with one
another, enquiring into the tastes, properties, forms, powers and names of all medicinal plants.

Having observed a plant with leaves dark-blue like
sapphire and with bulbs white like jasmine, crystal, the
white lotus, moonrays, or the conch shell, and having
his attention aroused by it, Susruta approached the sage
Kasiraja with the enquiry as to what it could be.

Kasiraja then tells the Indian story of the origin of
garlic. It begins with the legendary struggles between the
devas, gods of sweetness and light, and *asuras,* mischie-
vous demons. At an early period of time, the devas and
asuras made a truce and together churned the waters of
the Great Ocean—from this churning came the sun and
the moon, and also the amrita or elixir of immortality.
Rahu, king of the asuras, made off with the crystal vase
containing the elixir. The god Vishnu pursued him and
cut off his head. But from his throat, which had drunk
the elixir, drops fell to the ground—from these sprang
garlic. Other cultures have similar legends. There is a
Mohammedan story that, when Satan went from the
Garden of Eden, garlic appeared from the ground where
his left foot rested and onion appeared at his right.

There is indeed something heavenly and also demonic
about garlic. It gives food a divine flavor; it has healing
powers. On the other hand there have always been people
who find its pungent smell and taste unbearable. Its very
hellishness is the source of its strength. As we shall see, it
is the sulphur compounds which give it its pungency and
its active healing properties. It needs its demonic power.

Garlic, said the Bower manuscript, cures a long list of diseases: thinness, weakness of digestion, lassitude, coughs, colds in the head, inflammation of the skin, hemorrhoids, swelling of the abdomen, enlargement of the spleen, indigestion, acute abdominal pains, painful constipation, excessive flow of urine, excessive menstrual bleeding, worms, rheumatism, consumption, leprosy, epilepsy, and paralysis. It is an astonishing list—no wonder garlic was called a cure-all! Yet, wherever and whenever one looks, one finds very similar claims being made. With a few exceptions, we believe that they can be justified by the evidence we present in this book.

The Bower manuscript describes garlic as a bringer of joy and pleasure as well as health. The Festival of Garlic was observed when winter arrived and it was too cold for rooftop moonlit parties.

> Then on the housetops, gateways and upper windows, garlands of garlic richly set should be displayed, and on the ground itself one should have worship performed. One should also have the people of one's household wear wreaths of garlic. This is the manner of observing the festival, appointed for the people and known by the name of Svalpovama, the Incomparable.

2

Garlic Planted

Garlic grows in almost every part of the world, in temperate, subtropical and even tropical regions, and it will grow easily in your garden. You can give it a plot of its own or, even better, put it in among other plants. It will not take up a great deal of room above ground, as its main work is done below. Garlic is grown not from seed but from individual cloves. One clove, given the right conditions, will produce a bulb or head containing eight to twenty cloves, so it is a productive plant.

Garlic sends up a round, solid, smooth stem, which can grow up to one meter tall. The leaves, which are flattish, narrow, and about fifteen centimeters long, emerge from the bottom of the plant. A cluster of purple-white flowers grows out from the top of the stem, enclosed in a papery sheath. Garlic does not fertilize itself by pollination and cultivated plants rarely, if ever, produce seed.

Sickle-shaped garlic cloves are so familiar that they hardly need description. Is there a way of seeing them with a fresh eye? A medieval folktale collected by the Hebrew poet, Bialik, is about an island where garlic had never been seen before. The king's magician is given a clove:

> He took one of the cloves and tore off the covering with his thumbnail. He undressed her naked as on the day of her birth, the white line of her breasts, her secret flesh. Then the clove appeared in all her splendor, the one, the simple, the clear and the clean.

What can one add to that, except to say that the covering of garlic cloves is sometimes purple and also rather beautiful? Sometimes, the purple-clad cloves are stronger in flavor. By the way, do not worry if your cloves are comparatively small, as their flavor and goodness may be more concentrated. Cloves grown in good, organic soil are often smaller, but have been proved to contain a higher proportion of the flavor-producing and medicinal ingredients. They are also healthier and less prone to rot.

Garlic should be planted in late autumn for an early supply next year. If put in too early, it may start to come up before the winter and be killed later by frost. There is a tradition of planting garlic on the shortest day of the year. It can also be planted in the spring, for a later crop. Cloves should be put into the ground tip upwards at a depth of 5 cm (2 in). They should be spaced 20–25 cm (9 in) apart, with 30 cm (12 in) between rows. Garlic likes a reasonably dry and sunny location and a good but not over-fertilized soil. Sulphur and sulphides in the soil increase its potency and flavor.

Though garlic is the most famous of the plants which fight infections, it is troubled by certain ones itself. The best known of these is the black spotting of the skin and the rotting of cloves which occurs before and after har-

Figure 1: Garlic (*Allium Sativum*)

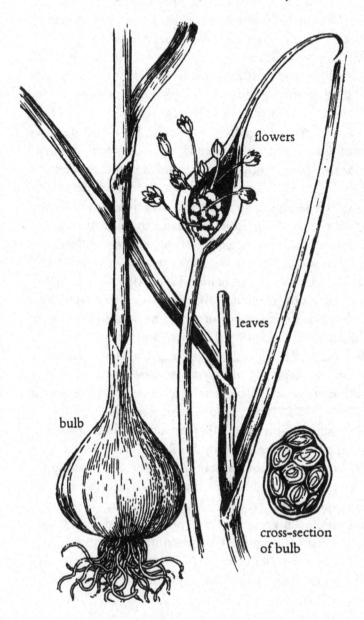

flowers

leaves

bulb

cross-section
of bulb

vest. This is caused by certain fungi called *Fusarium* and should be carefully watched for. In the ground, it may be attacked by mites, or tiny soil worms called nematodes.

As the plant matures, the stem, the leaves, and the roots all die away and it is then ready to harvest. This should be done during good weather. Pull up the bulb and remove the earth from it, then lay it out on the soil. It is essential to store garlic completely dry or rotting may occur. Garlic should be strung up in a cool, dry, and reasonably well-ventilated place and it will then keep for a year or more. Braiding bulbs together in decorative strings is a satisfying art. One can also tie them individually onto a piece of rope and hang them from that.

Garlic's botanical name is *Allium sativum*. *Allium* was the classical Latin name for garlic and *sativum* meant cultivated. The botanical name *Allium* describes a whole genus or group of plants. At one time, there were over 1,000 species of *Allium* but now the number has been reduced to around 450. The best known are the cultivated ones: the onion, *Allium cepa* (from the Latin for head); the leek, *Allium porrum;* the shallot, *Allium ascalonicum* (so called because it grew around Ascalon in Palestine); and chives, *Allium schoenoprasum.*

The alliums join the other groups of bulb plants to make up the Liliaceae or lily family, so garlic keeps company with that symbol of stainless purity. Also among the lilies are the daffodil, the tulip, the hyacinth, and the saffron-producing crocus. What distinguishes the alliums from other Liliaceae is their pungent and penetrating smell. What distinguishes them from underground vegetables of other families such as potatoes is that their bulbs are not part of their root systems but a continuation of their stems. This is most clearly observable with the leek, which is just a continuous tube. Whereas potatoes grow from the roots of the plant, and the turnip is just one giant root, garlic's tassel of rootlets grow out from below the bulb.

Many of the alliums are wild garlics. We have room to mention only a few of the more common ones. (See the table on page 13 for easy reference of common garlics.) *Allium ursinum,* ransoms or bear's garlic, carpets large areas in woods or river valleys. It likes moist, rich soil. It has broad elliptical leaves and beautiful clusters—called umbels—of white, star-shaped flowers. At first sight it can be mistaken for lily-of-the valley but as soon as you tread on it you know it is a garlic.

Allium scorodoprasum is the botanical name for rocambole or serpent garlic, whose central stem ends in marvelous snake-like twists and turns. It has purple flowers which later form a barb-shaped seed pod, giving the serpent a devil's tail. It has a small bulb which is mild and pleasant to the taste. Rocambole is sometimes called the sand leek, but this name properly belongs to *Allium ampeloprasum,* which grows wild in sandy regions and is considered to be the forerunner of the leek. It is also known as great-headed, elephant-headed, or giant garlic, since it grows up to 1.8 m (6 ft) in height, finally raising to the skies a large round ball of seeds. Its bulb sometimes, but not always, divides into cloves and has a mild, nutty flavor.

In the Far East, the alliums most commonly grown are *Allium fistulosum* (the Japanese bunching onion) and *Allium tuberosum* (*jiucai* or Chinese chives). The leaves of these plants are the mainstays of salads. Both are used medicinally; the great Chinese medical compendium, the *Ben Cao Gang Mu*, lists *jiucai* the first of all plants.

Allium vineale, or crow's garlic, grows wild in fields or on grassy banks. It has a 60 cm (2 ft.) long, spindly stem, hollow leaves, and small cloves the size of dried peas. Crow's garlic is supposed to have the ability to stupify those birds if they so much as land near it. So too does *Allium nothorscordum*, or false (non-smelling) garlic. We do not know if this phenomenon has ever been observed, but it adds a new dimension to the phrase "stone the crows."

Some alliums make good garden plants, having a delicate and unobtrusive beauty. *Allium flavum* looks nice in a rock garden and *Allium triquetum*, with its unusually shaped white flowers, is a good pot plant. *Allium moly*, with its bright yellow flowers, is another attractive garden plant. Its name derives from the moly of the Greek myths, being the herb which protected Odysseus from the spells of Circe and prevented her from turning him into a pig, as she had his sailors. Garlic is well known as a magical protector.

There are many interesting connections between garlic's various names. In ancient Mesopotamia it was known as *sum* or *shum*, the same as the modern Hebrew *shoum* and directly related to the Arabic *thoum*. Various derivations have been suggested for the Latin word allium. One is that it came from the word *halere*. As this means to give off a fragrant smell, perhaps a joke was intended. Whatever the odor, the Roman eagle carried it around the Mediterranean. The Latin *allium* became the Italian *aglio*, the French *ail*, and the Spanish *ajo*.

The ancient Greek name for garlic was *scorodon*. The famous French physician Henri Leclerc, who was a seri-

An Array of Alliums

Species	Common Name	Locality	Use
A. ampeloprasum	summer leek sand leek giant garlic	Europe Asia America	spice
A. ascalonicum	shallot	Europe Near East	vegetable spice remedy
A. bakeri	——	China Japan	vegetable spice remedy
A. cepa	onion	Europe Asia America	vegetable spice dye remedy
A. fistulosum	winter onion Japanese bunching onion	East Asia	spice remedy
A. flavum	yellow leek	Balkans Europe	ornamental
A. longiscuspis	original wild garlic	Turkestan	——
A. moly	yellow garlic	Europe	ornamental leaves as spice
A. nothorscordum	false garlic	Europe	——
A. porrum	leek	Europe Asia America	vegetable spice
A. schoenoprasum	chives	Europe Asia America	vegetable spice seeds as remedy
A. scorodoprasum	snake leek serpent garlic rocambole	Europe East Asia	spice
A. triquetum	——	East Medi- terranean	ornamental
A. tuberosum	Chinese chives	East Asia	vegetable
A. ursinum	wild garlic ransoms bear's garlic	Europe North Asia	remedy spice
A. vineale	crow's garlic	Europe	——

ous student of garlic and used it in his practice, derived it from *skaion rodon,* which he said meant *rose puante* or stinking rose. There is at present in California a society called "The Lovers of the Stinking Rose" which serves banquets, every course containing garlic.

The words *lauch, leac, luk* and so on are, in fact, common to many Germanic, Slavonic, and Celtic languages and mean either a leek or any kind of tasty plant. The English garlic comes directly from the Anglo-Saxon *garleac,* meaning spear-leek. It was known as the spear plant because of its flat, pointed leaves.

The Production Year Book of the Food and Agriculture Organization of the United Nations gives a world garlic crop of 2,315,000 metric tons. From this, one can estimate that, on average, each person in the world accounted for well over half a clove of garlic a day! Clearly garlic is spread world wide. The leading producers in 1982 were China, with an estimated 550,000 metric tons grown, and India, with an estimated 213,000 metric tons. The garlic specialists are also Spain with 197,000 metric tons in 1982, South Korea with 186,000 metric tons, Thailand with an estimated 180,000 metric tons, and Egypt with 166,000 metric tons. Egyptian fields gave by far the highest yield, with 33 metric tons per hectare, compared with a world average of just over six metric tons per hectare. This shows that garlic does well in hot, dry climates with plenty of irrigation.

The world is eating much more garlic. For example, over the last 25 years, garlic production has doubled in Spain, tripled in Egypt, Mexico, and Brazil and quadrupled in the United States, where most of the garlic is grown in and around the town of Gilroy, California.

3

Garlic Past

Garlic's first appearance in history is visual, not verbal, and takes us back nearly 6,000 years. In 1911, clay models of garlic bulbs were found in a tomb at El Mahasna in Egypt. They can be dated back to 3750 BC, well before the time of the Pharaohs. They were made of unbaked, whitewashed clay, with nine or more elongated rolls pressed around a globular core; experts have remarked on their lifelike quality.

In the tomb of the Pharaoh Tutankhamen, among the splendors of gold and lapis lazuli were found six garlic bulbs, dried and perfectly preserved. Garlic was found in many tombs. The tomb of the architect Kha, which dates from the same period, around 1500 BC, and which has been reassembled at the Egyptological Museum in Turin, was a simpler affair; it was like an ordinary room, with furniture, utensils, and various foodstuffs, including a basket of garlic. Why was it there? Did it have a religious or magical role as an offering to the gods or as a protector against evil? Was it sustenance for the soul on its journey to the halls of judgment?

Later Greek and Roman writers had some views about this. Pliny said that onions and garlic were sacred to the Egyptians because they swore oaths by them. Juvenal, who had an intense dislike of everything Egyptian, wrote in his fifteenth satire:

> *How Egypt mad with superstition grown*
> *Makes gods of monsters, but too well is known;*
> *Tis mortal sin an Onion to devour.*
> *Each clove of garlic has a sacred power.*
> *Religious nation, sure, and bless'd abodes*
> *Where every garden is o'er-run with gods.*

Whatever its place in religion, garlic was almost certainly a common item of Egyptian diet, in early times as it is now. The most famous garlic story of all concerns the amounts eaten by the builders of the Great Pyramid. We owe the story to the Greek historian, Herodotus, who visited Egypt around 450 BC. Recounting his visit to the Pyramid of Cheops at Giza he says:

> There is an inscription in Egyptian characters on the pyramid which records the quantity of radishes, onions and garlic consumed by the labourers who constructed it; and I perfectly well remember that the interpreter who read the writing to me said that the money expended in this way was sixteen thousand talents of silver.

It seems strange that such mundane information was inscribed on the walls of the Great Pyramid, which were used exclusively for religious texts. On the other hand, garlic would indeed have been an ideal and likely food for the workers; it would have been nutritious and would have protected them from disease.

We find a connection between garlic and Egyptian workers in the Bible. The Jews ate it when they were forced to labor for the Pharaohs of the New Kingdom 1,500 years later. They longed for it during their forty years wandering the desert:

> Then the rabble who had joined the people were over-come by greed, and the Sons of Israel began to wail again, "Who will give us meat to eat?" They said, "Think of the fish we used to eat free in Egypt, the cucumbers, melons, leeks, onions and garlic! Here we are, wasting away, stripped of everything; there is nothing but manna for us to look at." (Numbers 11: 4-6)

Once settled in Canaan, the Jews resumed their garlic eating and have continued it ever since. The Talmud recommends that it should be eaten especially on the eve of the Sabbath, in order to encourage the matrimonial love-making appropriate to that day.

Garlic has always been popular in the Middle East and the earliest civilizations of Mesopotamia grew and ate it. Texts dating from the reign of King Naram-Sin, who ruled from 2260–2233 BC, show *sum* being distributed to important individuals, to lords, generals, and governors. There was often a considerable volume of trade; one account, dating from the time of King Nabonidus, who yielded the throne of Babylon to Cyrus in 538 BC, mentions the transfer of no less than 150,000 strings of garlic: fifteen million bulbs!

Garlic was found when the palace at Knossos was excavated. We know that the Athenians of the Classical Age reveled in their garlic. It was a common item of diet and renowned for giving health and energy. Aristotle described it as a tonic. On new moon nights, the Greeks used to leave out banquets of garlic for Hecate, the Queen of the Underworld. These were placed on piles of stones at crossroads. Garlic's link with darkness and the depths is worldwide, but has always been particularly strong in Greece and the Balkans; here we have early evidence of it.

The plays of the ancient Greek playwright Aristophanes are full of jokes about garlic. Some are medical, so his audience must have been thoroughly familiar with its medical uses. Someone hobbling uncomfortably along in a pair of new boots is told that he looks as if he is curing a boil on his foot with a clove of garlic. When others of Aristophanes' characters eat garlic, they become aggressive and warlike, and he records that it even played a part in starting the Peloponnesian War:

> Some drunken young fellows stole a girl named Simathia,
> so the Megarians, primed with garlic, stole two girls of
> Aspasia's in revenge, and with that began the war which
> broke out all over Greece.

Of course there will always be those who do not like to be too close to the smell of garlic on someone else's breath. In Aristophanes' play *Thesmophoriazusae,* we learn how this can be used to establish an alibi. Certain young women have taken to deceiving their soldier husbands who are on night-sentry duty. Coming back at dawn, they quickly eat cloves of garlic so that their husbands will never imagine that they have been unfaithful.

The Romans, like the Greeks, valued garlic for the strength it gave their soldiers. Indeed, garlic and soldiering were synonymous; *allia ne comedas,* "may you not eat garlic," was the Roman equivalent of "may you not receive your draft papers." The Romans were extremely efficient in supplying their legions with food and medical supplies and garlic was certainly carried by the Romans to the borders of their Empire, to France, to Spain, and to England. There they planted it, together with the violet and the rose, beneath the walls of their forts and in the gardens of their villas.

Garlic was also the food of Roman farmers and farm laborers. The poet Virgil describes it as "essential to maintain the strength of harvesters." Here he depicts the height of the harvest season:

> *Now even the cattle seek the cool shade,*
> *Now the green lizards hide in the thorn thickets,*
> *And Thestylis pounds for the reapers, spent with the scorching*
> *Heat, her savoury herbs of garlic and thyme.*

Strangely, the Romans also condemned criminals to a daily diet of it, *pro criminum expiatione aliis*. However, there may have been a quasi-magical side to this; purity rather than punishment may have been intended, since pungent smells have often been used in rites of purification. In England, too, at a time when medicine and magic were close, we find garlic as first line protection against both. In a collection of remedies written out for a doctor named Bald, around AD 900, we find the following (recorded in an 1865 book, *Leechdoms, Wortcunning and Starcraft of Early England*):

> Work thus a salve against the elfin race and nocturnal goblin visitors, and for women with whom the devil

hath commerce: take the female hop plant, wormwood, bishopwort, lupin, ashthroat, henbane, harewort, viper's bugloss, heathberry plants, cropleek garlic, grain of hedgerife, githrife, fennel: put these worts into a vessell, set them under the altar, sing over them nine masses, boil them in butter and sheep's grease, add much holy salt, strain through a cloth, and throw the worts into running water.

Those at risk had the ointment rubbed on their foreheads, eyes, and body; they were censed with incense and had the sign of the cross made over them. Of course, Bald's book also has some useful garlic remedies for more ordinary complaints, such as coughs and swellings; we give one of them in our last chapter.

At some time, garlic fell out of favor with the English and with English-speaking people. It remained out of favor for a long time and their prejudice against it is only just now coming to an end. When did it begin? Shakespeare's references to garlic indicate a lowly role for it. It is the food of rustics (*Henry IV*, Parts I; III, 1 and *A Winter's Tale* IV, 3), common working men (*Midsummer Night's Dream* IV, 2 and *Coriolanus* IV, 6) and beggars (*Measure for Measure* III, 2). Yet we believe that Shakespeare was secretly on garlic's side. In *Midsummer Night's Dream,* Bottom the weaver tells his fellow actors to "eat no onions or garlic, for we are to utter sweet breath." Yet it is the garlic-eating Bottom who is loved by Titania, and attended by her fairies.

Clearer signs of the prejudice can be seen during the seventeenth century. The herbalists, for the first time, begin to apologize for garlic's smell. The famous herbalist Culpeper in 1649 spoke of "the offensiveness of the breath of him that hath eaten garlick." John Evelyn, diarist and writer on many branches of natural history, summed up the new view in his *Acetaria, a Discourse of Sallets* (or salads), published in 1699. Spaniards and Italians, he says, eat it with everything. It is known as a medicine and it is all right for country people, especially if they live in damp places, or for seamen, but

> . . . we absolutely forbid its entrance into our Salleting, by reason of its intolerable Rankness, and which made it so detested of old: that the eating of it was (as we read) part of the Punishment for such as had committed the horrid'st crimes. To be sure 'tis not for Ladies Palats, nor those who court them, further than to permit a light touch on the Dish, with a clove there of, much better supply'd by the gentler Rocambo.

And the poet Shelley on a visit to France wrote back:

> What do you think? Young women of rank eat—you will never guess what—garlick!

There was thus a division between the English, and also other northern European races like the Germans, and the peoples of the Mediterranean; the one may have linked garlic to the indiscipline and hot blood of the other. "Unless very sparingly used," says Mrs. Beeton, in her cookbook that was the bible of Victorian households, "the flavor is disagreeable to the English palate."

The difference of view spread to the English colonies—and to the countries of the New World. A United States Department of Agriculture pamphlet of 1938 remarked that "demand is practically limited to the needs of the Mediterranean races, the main markets being New York, Chicago and St. Louis."

Since that time, however, the whole situation has changed. After World War II, foreign travel became much more common and foreign cooking more appreciated. New generations of English and white Americans have begun to shake themselves free of the age-old prejudice. Garlic has even attained something of a cult status in California and the annual garlic festival at Gilroy, near San Francisco, now rivals those of Spain and southern France. We hope that, in the end, everyone will realise how tasty it is, and how beneficial to health. Its pungency will then present no problems, for garlic eaters never notice the smell of garlic, either on themselves or on others.

Whether they eat it or not, everyone knows one thing about garlic: it keeps off vampires. Bram Stoker's famous book *Dracula* is the usual source of this knowledge; when bulbs were placed on the heroine's window sill, the blood-sucking Count could not pass. Stoker was in fact drawing on age-old traditions and no book about garlic would be complete without some account of them. The belief that it protects against misfortune and the evil eye is found in almost every part of the world. However, its connection with vampires seems to belong almost exclusively to Eastern Europe and the Balkans and it is in those regions that we find the richest store of customs, many of which are still alive today. There, garlic's help was called on at every crucial stage of life, when harm might befall. Women put it on their pillows during childbirth and in their children's clothes at baptism. If a child would not take its mother's milk, its lips were smeared with garlic. Young men about to be married kept away evil spirits with it; brides braided it in their hair. The gypsies even put it into the coffins of the dead, thus ensuring the soul's eternal life.

The author Phillip Thornton tells this story in his autobiographical book *Iron and Oxen,* published in 1939. While staying in a small village in the Carpathian mountains in northern Romania, he was invited to the funeral of a young child. Here he is describing the burial:

> The two boys in charge of the bier carried it to within a yard of the open grave and then removed the coffin lid. The priest, vested in a faded purple chasuble, blessed the grave, cutting the sign of the cross into the earth with a spade. Then he aspersed the dead child twice with water and once with oil, crossing the forehead with his thumb. The mother filled the child's mouth with garlic and drew the shroud over the little creature's head. She also placed a ten lei coin in the child's right hand, for the ferry fare across the Styx. The lid was replaced and the father lowered the coffin into the grave with a length of lines.

Thornton was told how the child had been found dead in a garden adjoining the parent's house, the victim of a vampire. On the occasion quoted above, the garlic would have been used to keep the soul of the dead child from harm and most of all, to prevent the vampire from making further use of the body as a base for its activities. Is it effective against such monsters? We would firmly wish not to have the opportunity of finding out.

In the countries of the Orient, garlic was also used against the evil eye, but the priesthood didn't necessarily get along with it. Garlic is almost universally used in

India, however the Laws of Manu forbade Brahmins to eat it. And today, garlic may not be brought to certain pilgrimage places, such as Gangotri near the source of the Ganges. The Bower manuscript proposed a way around the prohibition: feed a cow with garlic for three days and a Brahmin may drink her milk. In fact, now it is only the strictly celibate yogis and a few Jains and Brahmins who keep the rule, on the grounds that garlic would stimulate their passions. One of the authors of this book found this out when he was staying in Benares. As a friendly gesture he offered some garlic to an elderly Indian neighbor of his; unfortunately the old man was a lifelong celibate and chased him angrily out of his room.

It is recorded that the Buddha's most senior disciple, Sariputra, cured himself of an upset stomach by eating garlic; thus Buddhist monks are allowed it as a medicine. However, they are not officially allowed it as a food for fear of upsetting the other monks. The rule which reached Tibet was even stricter: if you have eaten garlic, you may not enter your monastery even to save it from burning down. However, we have it on first-hand authority that this was a prohibition which Tibetan monks generally ignored, sensibly in view of the cold climate.

In Japan likewise, Zen Buddhist temples had notices at their gates saying that alchohol and "kun" (meaning all vegetables of the onion class) could not be brought inside; in country areas these notices could still be seen quite recently. Buddhism came to Japan in the sixth century AD and, at that time, the Japanese adopted a new word for garlic, *ninniku,* the characters for which mean "to bear insults with patience." The Japanese have never been great garlic eaters, perhaps because the Koreans, to whom they consider themselves superior, eat such a lot of it. In this, they differ from the Ainu, the aboriginal people of Sakhalin, the northernmost island of the Japanese archipelago. They believe that wild garlic is the food of their gods. When a child is born, and the family gather round to celebrate, they throw it into the fire to summon the gods to attend the festival.

With that far distant ceremonial we must end this brief account of man's relationship with garlic. We have considered his likes and dislikes, his prayers and rituals, but we have as yet said little about garlic's traditional role as a medicine. We deal with this wide-ranging topic in our next chapter.

4

Garlic Prescribed

For the thousands of years of man's history, medicine meant herbal medicine. The changeover to chemically defined and synthetically produced medicines began during the twentieth century. Until then it was plants, eaten raw, dried, steeped, brewed, or cooked, which provided man with his remedies, together with a lesser number of animal substances and some naturally-occuring minerals. Garlic has always had an honorable place among medicinal plants. Wherever one looks, one finds its uses described in a remarkably consistent way.

Let us begin in ancient Greece; having mentioned some Greek jokes about garlic, let us now take the subject seriously. The Greeks' most famous physician was Hippocrates, who lived from 460–370 BC and is known as the Father of Medicine; he founded a medical school on the Aegean island of Kos. Hippocrates and other Greek doctors are a mine of information on our subject. Garlic was used, first of all, as a cleanser of the digestive system and as a diuretic.

> It is good for increasing the flow of urine. It is best taken
> when one is about to drink too much, or when one is
> drunk. Garlic boiled or roasted is a diuretic, and relaxes
> the stomach.
>
> Garlic causes flatulence, because it stops flatulence.

The last is an example of the Hippocratic principle of
curing like by like.

Diocles prescribed a clove of garlic placed inside a fig
as a digestive purge, "a more efficient one being fresh
garlic taken in neat wine with coriander." Praxagoras
mixed it with oil in stew for severe bowel pains.

Secondly, it was used for dealing with infections and
inflammations of various kinds, internal and external—
for example, of the lung. Again, from Hippocrates:

> But if there is no cough and you recognise the signs of
> suppuration, the sick man, for his evening meal and
> before he goes to bed, should eat raw garlic in great
> quantity and should drink a noble and pure wine. If by
> this means the pus erupts, so much the better. For in-
> flammation of the rectum, one uses a poultice of garlic
> cooked in black wine mixed with water.

Hippocrates also used garlic to encourage menstruation, to bring away the afterbirth, and in the following
pregnancy test:

> To know whether a woman will bear a child. Clean a
> clove of garlic, cut off the top, place it in the vagina and
> see if next day her mouth smells of it. If she smells, she
> will conceive; if not, she will not.

It was in Roman times that the foundations of Western

medicine were established. The most influential writer on herbs was Dioscorides, who lived in the first century AD. He was a Greek, and chief physician to the Roman armies in Asia Minor. His *Materia Medica* gives the following account of garlic's virtues and vices.

> Garlic is sharp, biting, wind producing, excites the belly, and creates thirst. If eaten it helps eliminate the tapeworm, it drives out the urine. It is good against snake bite with wine, or when crushed with wine. It is good against the bite of a rabid dog. It makes the voice clear, and soothes continuous coughing when eaten raw or boiled. Boiled with oregano, it kills lice and bed bugs. It clears the arteries. Burnt and mixed with honey, it is an ointment for blood-shot eyes; it also helps baldness. Together with salt and oil, it heals eczema. Together with honey, it heals white spots, herpetic eruptions, liver spots, leprosy and scurvy. Boiled with pine-wood and incense, it soothes toothache when the solution is kept in the mouth. Boiling the umbrel of the flowers is good for a sitting bath to help the coming of menstruation and the placenta. For the same purposes it can be smoked. A mush from crushed garlic and black olives is a diuretic. It is helpful in dropsy (edema).

Another notable authority was Gaius Pliny the Elder. His *Natural History* runs to many volumes and covers a vast range of subjects. Here is a part of what he says on garlic:

> Garlic is believed to be useful for making a number of medicaments, especially those used in the country. . . . For the bites of serpents it is very efficacious to roast it with its own leaves and make a linament by adding oil; also for bruises on the body, even if they have swollen

into blisters . . . . To asthmatics it is given cooked, though some have given it raw. Pounded and drunk with vinegar and water, it is useful as a gargle for boils in the throat. By three pounded heads with vinegar tooth-ache is relieved, as it is by rinsing the teeth with a decoction, and inserting garlic itself into the hollow tooth. Garlic juice, mixed with goose grease, is also dropped into the ears. Garlic in drink, or infused with vinegar and nitrum, checks lice and scurf, it stops catarrhs if boiled with milk, also beaten up and mixed with soft cheese . . . . For a cough a decoction is taken with stale grease, or with milk; or if there be also spitting of blood or pus, it is roasted under live ashes and taken with an equal part of honey. With fat, it cures suspected tumours. Mixed with sulphur and resin it draws the pus from fistulas [pipe-shaped ulcers or infections], with pitch extracting even arrows. Leprous sores, and lichen-like and freckly eruptions are cleansed and cured by it and wild marjoram, or by a linament made of its ash with oil and fish sauce. Used in this way it is also good for erisypelas [inflammations of the skin, deep red in colour]. One head of it taken in dry wine with an obolus [$\frac{1}{6}$ of a drachma] of silphium shakes off malaria . . . . It induces sleep also, and makes the body of a ruddier colour. It is believed to act as an aphrodisiac, when pounded with fresh coriander and taken with neat wine. It injures the stomach when taken too freely and creates thirst.

Garlic was certainly being used for a considerable num-ber of conditions. It is not surprising that Galen, the most influential doctor of all time, having seen a countryman eat it and cure himself instantly of bowel pains, called it *theriacum rusticorum*. Countryman's cure-all would be a good translation, since a *theriacum* was a remedy for all complaints.

How could there be any sense in such a variety of uses?

Yet, if one examines them carefully, a pattern does emerge. Firstly, garlic helps digestion and elimination. Edema and swellings are caused by poor functioning of the kidneys, or by poor blood circulation, which garlic also helps ("it clears the arteries"). It acts against various kinds of inflammations and infections, including coughs, respiratory problems, and even tuberculosis ("spitting of blood or pus"). It is an anti-toxin for poisonous bites and stings and it kills internal parasites. It gives energy; we have already seen that the Greeks and Romans regarded it as a general tonic. At the same time, garlic can have adverse effects; it can irritate the stomach or the skin. If one looks at the list of uses given in the Bower manuscript, one finds that they are very similar and, throughout history, the same claims continue to be made with remarkable consistency.

The medical practices of the Romans passed chiefly to the Arabs, and the great Arab doctors, such as Avicenna, used garlic. So too did the medieval medical school of Salerno, in Sicily. Another of garlic's medieval champions was that remarkable woman St. Hildegarde of Bremen, who was born in 1099. Despite being a cloistered nun and a recognized visionary, she was one of the foremost writers of her age on botany and other scientific topics. Indeed, as a nun (and later an abbess) she would have been concerned with health and healing, since it was to the religious houses that many, especially the poor, came for treatment. Of garlic she said:

> It gives health both to those who are well and those who are ill. And it ought to be eaten raw, because if it is cooked, its strength is lost. Neither does it hurt the eyes, nor on account of its heat is the blood around the

eyes strongly excited by it, but through it they become clear.

Here Hildegard is refuting the widespread belief, dating from Hippocratic times, that garlic is bad for the eyes; it is difficult to account for especially as, unlike onion, garlic does not make you cry when you cut it. St. Hildegarde continues:

> It should be eaten in moderation, lest the blood of a man overheats. In truth, if garlic is forbidden, a man's health and proper strength vanish away; but if it is then mixed with food in due proportion, it will bring back his strength.

With the Renaissance came a flowering of medical and botanical studies. The first substantial herbal in English was William Turner's *New Herbal* of 1562. Turner spent some time in exile for his extreme Protestant views, but Queen Elizabeth I gave him her special protection and he became her herbalist. "Garleke," he said, "is hote and drye in the fourth degree." This is according to the Galenical classification of medicines which have four qualities (hot, dry, moist and cold) in four degrees of strength, the fourth being the most powerful. Garlic, being hot and dry and full of rising movement, is good at combating moist and cold diseases, and this matches perfectly with its power to break up catarrh and bronchial congestion and to clear away impurities in the digestion and the blood.

In 1649 the London College of Physicians valued garlic as an antidote to poisons and to the bites of venomous beasts, as an encourager of urine and bowel movements, and as good for edema, ulcers, and toothache. They used it only as a "simple," that is to say on its own and not in their elaborate mixtures. We know this because the young and independently-minded doctor, Nicholas Culpeper, translated their official pharmacopeia from Latin into English and used it as the basis of his own herbal. Culpeper added an astrological ascription: "Mars owns this herb." If one is going to link plants and planets, Mars seems the appropriate one for garlic, since both are bringers of dynamic energy. (Enthusiastic astrologers might like to plant their garlic on 6th or 7th November, at 15° Scorpio.) Later editions of Culpeper's herbal contained the following warning.

> Garlic's heat is very vehement, and everything of that description naturally conveys ill-humours to the brain. In choleric cases it adds fuel to the fire; in men oppressed with melancholy it extenuates the humor, and confounds the idea with strange visions and fancies.

The advice not to use garlic in "choleric cases" implies not to use it during hot inflammation or fever. It might also exaggerate the aggressiveness of those inclined to anger; the ancient Greeks certainly believed as much. However, as to "strange visions and fancies," in no way, we are sure, is garlic an hallucinogen!

Garlic was one of the many remedies suggested by the College of Physicians for the Great Plague of London in 1665. There is a tale that it then cost a guinea an ounce and that no one who ate it died. Whatever the truth of this, garlic has often had the reputation of being able to protect against the plague. In Marseilles in 1721, so the story runs, four thieves were released from prison in order to collect and bury the bodies of the victims of the plague which was then raging. Such workers were not expected to live long, but to everyone's surprise, the four remained healthy. It was then discovered that they were drinking vinegar mixed with garlic juice every day. From that time on "Four Thieves Vinegar", *"Vinaigre des Quatres Voleurs,"* was sold in Marseilles; in our last chapter we give the recipe for it.

John Waller, author of the *New British Domestic Herbal* of 1822, observed a similar occurrence during a plague in Oxford.

> The author can vouch for the circumstances that, during the prevalance of a very contagious fever in the vicinity of Somers Town and St. Giles, the French ecclesiastics who constantly used the plant in all their culinary preparations visited the most filthy and infectious hovels with impunity, whilst the English ministers of the same religion were generally infected with the contagion, to which several of them fell victim.

In all these cases, garlic might have given internal protection against infection and it might also have discouraged the plague-carrying fleas from biting, for it has often been said that insects do not care for garlicky blood.

It is surprising to learn how often garlic has been used against serious illness, and with some success. Sir Thomas Sydenham (1624-1689), one of the founding fathers of English medicine, described how he used it as part of his treatment for smallpox and how he cured a young nobleman in this way. In the medical journals of Paris between 1849 and 1853, three reports appeared of effective treatments of cholera in Provence and elsewhere. Poultices and massages with infusions of garlic were used. Nearer our own time, Dr. Albert Schweitzer is reported to have used garlic against cholera and typhoid in his mission hospital in Africa.

Garlic continued to be widely used by doctors in England until the second half of the nineteenth century. Jonathan Stoke's *A Botanical Materia Medica* of 1812 lists comments about garlic appearing in no less than forty medical books of the time. It was called a tonic, a diuretic (to promote urination), a stomachic, an expectorant (to clear the lungs and throat), a febrifuge (to reduce fevers), a diaphoretic or sudorific (to produce sweating), an antihelminthic (to remove and kill worms), a rubefacient (to cause irritation or burning on the skin), and as an emmenagogue (to regulate menstruation): the traditional uses under new names. However, the tide was turning against plant medicines, and garlic, because of its smell, was probably among the first to lose popularity. An article in *The Practitioner* in 1870 listed it among "the quaint and absurd medicaments . . . now obsolete among physicians." In the United States, the old-style country physician, who used local folk remedies along with the more modern drugs, survived longer than in Britain. Herbal medicine also lasted more successfully on the continent of Europe, through the tradition of health spas and natural cures.

In other parts of the world, and especially among poorer people, garlic has never lost its place as an important medicine. Because it is so easily available and covers so many conditions, it is the typical folk remedy. Here are a few instances, out of many. In Iran, people chew cloves to keep away coughs and influenza. The Druze, in the hilly areas of Lebanon and Israel, give women great quantities of garlic for ten days after childbirth in order to prevent infections and bring the uterus back to shape. Gypsies everywhere use it, especially crushed in milk, for all kinds of children's ailments. In Majorca, a garlic "cure" is commonly taken in autumn: one clove every day before breakfast for one week, two cloves a day in the second week, three cloves in the third, two cloves in the fourth, and in the fifth week again one clove daily. This is designed to keep away colds, coughs, and rheumatic problems during the coming winter. In the USSR, garlic is highly regarded. Paul Kourenoff, in his *Russian Folk Medicine*, describes how it is used to build up strength and improve the circulation of the elderly: minced garlic and onion are mixed with apple vinegar and honey to make a syrup. Another Russian remedy uses 450 grams of garlic ground with the juice of twenty-four lemons; this is left for three weeks, then a teaspoonful taken daily for obesity in old people and for general debility. European household tips include applying crushed garlic to bites and stings and a sliver in the cheek for toothache or in the ear for ear infections. Garlic syrups for coughs are common. These syrups are made by crushing garlic in honey, perhaps because honey is both nutritious and antiseptic and also can help disguise garlic's taste and smell.

In the Orient, herbal medicine is still officially recognized; it never lost its strength and sophistication as it did in the West. In India, the Ayurvedic tradition is still widely practiced and garlic is used much as it was at the time of the Bower manuscript. In China, herbs, together with acupuncture, massage, and other traditional therapies take their place alongside conventional modern medicine. Patients in clinics and hospitals are treated with one or the other, according to their own preferences and the nature of their problems. The Chinese look on garlic as a pungent herb, warming in quality. It is not one of the gentle "kingly" herbs, which are only used preventatively, to balance and adjust the body's processes. It is a non-toxic, middle-range remedy, both curative and preventive. It is to some extent too strong in flavor and action for the Chinese, who prefer to use the gentler *Allium fistulosum* or *Allium tuberosum* for the same purposes. Its principle use in Chinese herbalism is as an antidote to intestinal worms. A modern Chinese herbal manual gives the following uses for garlic, which by now should sound familiar.

- For dysentery: eat fresh garlic and take a garlic-juice enema.
- For resolving boils and carbuncles: a garlic plaster with oil.
- For whooping cough, tuberculosis, and coughs: garlic taken with other herbs.
- For insect and snake bites: apply crushed garlic to the bite. Also boil garlic and *Sophora subrostata* (a Chinese herb) and take internally.
- For helping the flow of urine and resolving edema: take garlic and plantain.

Herbalism in the West, having declined almost to extinction, is now enjoying a revival, and there are now many practicing herbalists. We spoke to herbalist Dr. Malcolm Stuart, who runs the Cambridge Herb Clinic, about garlic. He gives fresh extracts for bronchial infections, laryngitis, and tonsillitis, sometimes as a gargle with myrrh; also for ulcers, abscesses, and septicemia. He also uses it to lower blood pressure and to help against hardening of the arteries. Like the Russians, he finds it effective for the general debility which can affect the elderly; for this he mixes it with damiana, kola, centaury, and other herbs. Like the Chinese, he regards it as "strong" medicine and therefore one of the herbs closest to drugs as they are understood by the modern medical establishment. On the occasions that his patients find it upsetting to their digestion, he mixes it with stomach-calming herbs like sweet-flag, angelica, fennel, or dill.

We have so far said nothing about garlic for animals, but it works as well for them as it does for human beings, and for the same kinds of conditions. The European country folk who hung garlic on the doors of their barns and on the horns of their cattle to guard against misfortune also put it in their animals' feed to keep them healthy. While researching this book, we visited a farmer, Mr. Arthur Oaks, who keeps sheep and horses on the edge of Exmoor, in Devon, England. Twenty years ago, on the advice of a local gypsy renowned for his knowledge of animals, he began giving garlic to his sheep against influenza and found it extremely effective. He has also kept his animals free from worms by giving the horses a three-month course of garlic tablets during the winter, and the sheep raw garlic juice with root of male fern and couch grass; he finds he needs no other kind of worm treatment and the worms never become resistant.

Having begun this chapter far back in time, let us end on a personal, present-day note. The cat belonging to one of the authors of this book was recently very ill; she refused food and water for five days and was at death's door. Finally—something that should have been done before—she was given a few spoonfuls of crushed garlic in milk. She revived immediately, began to eat and was soon quite recovered.

In this chapter, we have tried to show the unity behind the diverse uses of garlic as a medicine. However, any attempt to bring it into the modern age must take into account the scientific research which checks the ancient traditions. Can garlic stand the test?

5

Garlic Probed

The search for the chemical constituents of plant medicines began in earnest around the beginning of the nineteenth century. There were several early successes; morphine was extracted from the opium poppy in 1803 and cinchona bark gave up its quinine soon after. Garlic, too, was mashed, heated, distilled, acidified, and mixed with alkalis. The concentrated and powerful oil which emerged from such operations was used medicinally, but no great progress was made in determining its chemistry. It was observed that it contained sulphur—not a difficult conclusion given the fumes that must have filled the laboratories; however, sulphur is a very common constituent of organic matter.

The first significant observations were made by Professor Wertheim in 1844. By condensing the steam which he passed through a bubbling garlic mush, he produced what he called "an evil-smelling oil" whose main component was, he said, diallyl sulphide. He coined the word allyl from the *Allium* of garlic, and it is now in regular usage in chemistry. Professor Wertheim was nearly there: on the right track but at the last moment caught the wrong culprit. It was not until 1892 that A.P. Semmler correctly identified the main components of garlic oil. The major one, which had garlic's characteristic smell and made up 60% of the total contents, was diallyl disulphide. He also found diallyl trisulphide (20%) and several other sulphur compounds.

There was one mystery, among many. How does garlic come to taste and smell as it does? In its natural state, it is quite odor free. A peeled whole clove, uncut, doesn't taste or smell. If you boil a whole head uncut and untouched, you get a vegetable taste, somewhere between onion, mustard, and potato. It is sharply pungent only after it has been bruised or crushed. In 1944, the scientists Cavallito, Bailey, and Buck, who were working for the Winthrop Chemical Company in the United States, got part of the way toward a solution. Using the most sophisticated techniques of the time, including spectroscopic analysis, they found that undamaged garlic tissue contains a certain mysterious sulphur compound which has no taste or smell. When garlic is cut or crushed, this original and as yet unknown material somehow produces a highly reactive and pungent new compound which they identified for the first time. In chemical terms it was diallyl thiosulphinate, commonly known as *allicin*. They had found the active component of garlic, and soon proved that it was a powerful bacteria-killer. Yet allicin is too reactive to last long. It is unstable, and in a few days changes itself into the strong smelling oily sulphur compounds like diallyl disulphide, that are the main constituents of garlic oil.

The complete picture emerged through the researches of two Swiss chemists, Dr. Arthur Stoll and Dr. Ewald Seebeck. By crushing garlic at a very low temperature, they were actually able to extract the mysterious forerunner of allicin just as it exists inside garlic. They carefully purified it and eventually succeeded in isolating crystals of a sulphur-rich amino acid which they called alliin. The substance which changes alliin into allicin they found to be an enzyme (i.e. a natural biological catalyst made from protein), which they called allinase. Alliin and allinase exist separately in the cell until crushing of some kind brings them together and the chain reaction is set in motion.

Alliin, as we said, is an amino acid. Amino acids are present in the body in considerable quantities; twenty of them are the building blocks from which the proteins of all living organisms are made. One of these, called cysteine, contains sulphur. The common cysteine helps to make all kinds of rather special sulphur-containing amino acids in garlic, leek, chives, onion, and even in cabbage and mustard. All of them have strong flavors and quite a strong influence on us humans. They form, for example, the substances in onions that make us cry as well as the ones in garlic that make us well.

Figure 2 shows the script of garlic's chemical drama. The chemical formulas of these unusual compounds are given in Figure 3.

Garlic has another chemical act we should know about. Professor Erick Block of New York State University at Albany found that when garlic was heated with water and solvents such as acetone in the laboratory, the allicin goes in another direction—to make a compound called

Figure 2: Transformation of Garlic's Active Ingredients

Normal amino acid

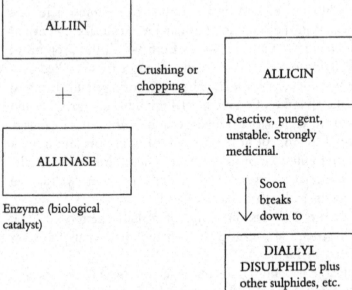

Special garlic amino acid: no taste or smell; no medicinal action.

Enzyme (biological catalyst)

Main constituents of garlic oil: strong smell and taste; medicinally active.

Figure 3: Chemical Structure of Garlic's Active Ingredients

Cysteine

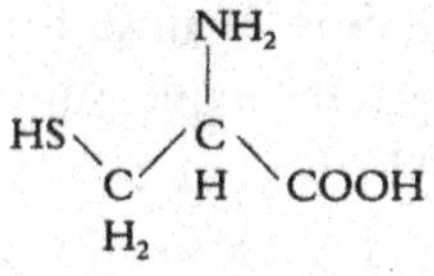

Alliin

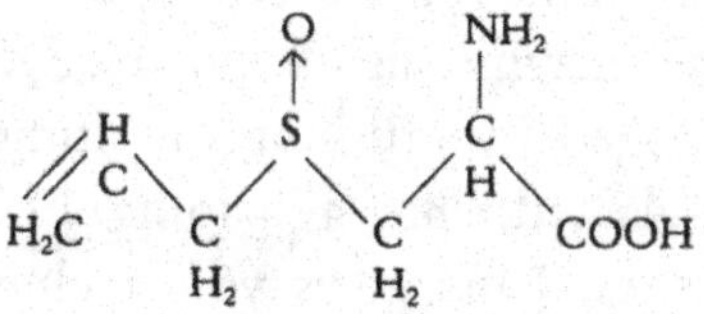

Allicin

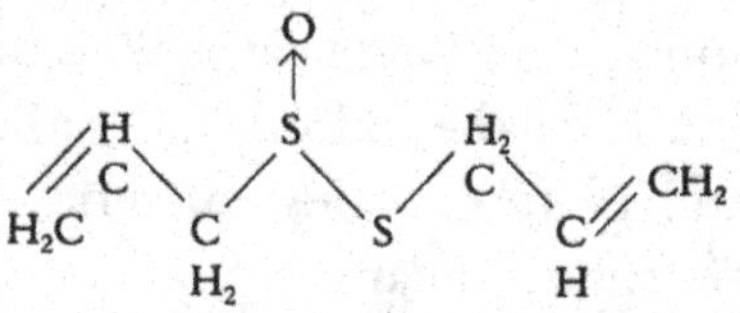

Diallyl Disulphide

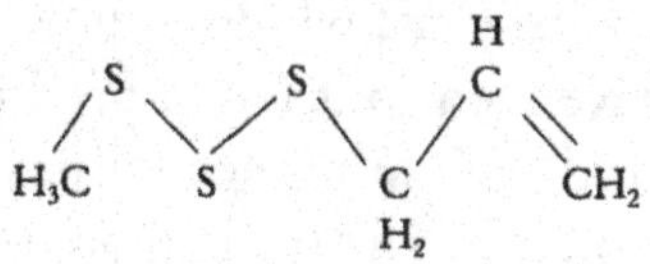

Methyl Allyl Trisulphide (Example of another oil constituent)

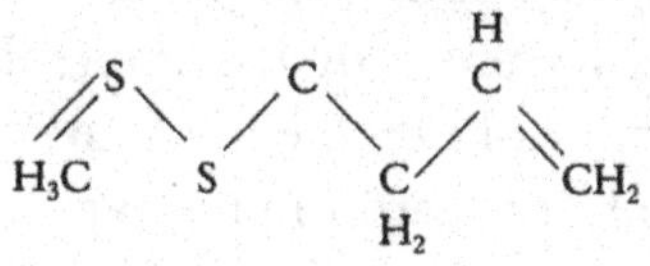

Ajoene

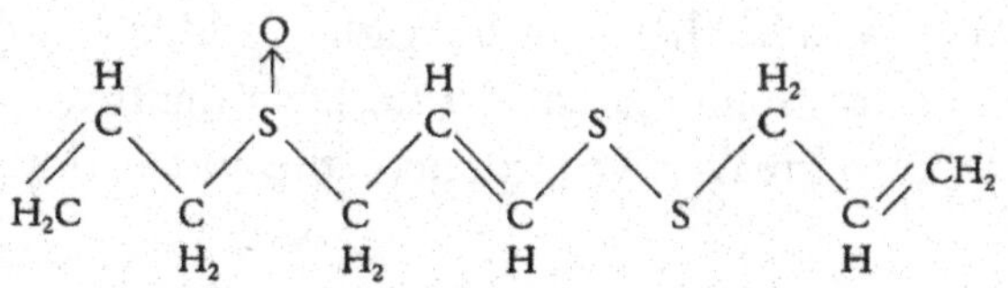

ajoene (from the Spanish ajo, meaning garlic). This is a very potent medicine against blood clotting which researchers are currently exploring as a basis for new anti-clotting drugs. However it may be a product of the laboratory only, as it does not appear in natural garlic whether cooked, crushed or dried.

Dissolved in the fluids of the cell, alliin waits. In another section, the enzyme also stands ready. As soon as the cells are damaged by crushing or biting, the allicin powerhouse is released, like a flaming Phoenix rising from the cold ashes. This gives you a clue as to why garlic does this. Imagine the shock facing any animal, insect, or worm that takes a bite out of garlic. Allicin is garlic's protection against being eaten by pests just as the crying compound is for the onion. And garlic's defensive substances defend us too, against bacteria, worms, and other "pests" affecting humans.

As soon as allicin is made, it begins bit by bit to decay. The major products are diallyl disulphide and diallyl trisulphide, as we have seen. But it also produces a whole range of other kinds of sulphides, disulphides, and trisulphides such as methyl allyl trisulphide, thiols such as methanethiol, and other compounds. This oily "soup" is very strong smelling and tasting and is the typical garlicky odor. As allicin decays more or less immediately if it is cooked or fried after crushing, the fried garlic is therefore equivalent to this oil. It is hard to preserve the allicin and stop it from turning into the oil. Vitamin C, citrus oils, and low temperature help preserve it. However, it still decays, and therefore all garlic products and garlic that you crush and eat are an unstable mixture of allicin and its oily breakdown products, the proportions depending on how they are treated. Heated garlic and garlic oil capsules will have gone all the way to the oil, while freshly crushed garlic will contain almost all of the original allicin. It makes a difference to us since allicin and the oily compounds have different effects on the body.

Diallyl disulphide and the other components of the oil also change and become, in time, an exotic mixture of di-, tri- and polysulphides and other similar materials. Sulphides generally have strong smells, but it is the simpler sulphides which have the stronger smells; the smell of rotten eggs is due to a gas, hydrogen sulphide, which is the simplest of all and, fortunately, is not present in garlic. Most of the polysulphides which are among the final breakdown products of allicin are not effective as medicines and have little smell or taste. In other words, extracts lose their strength after weeks or months of storage, faster if they are heated or if they are left exposed to the air.

The amounts of active constituents present are by no means constant, but vary according to the location and methods of cultivation. Alliin and sulphur content run roughly parallel, and Stoll and Seebeck found enormous variation in sulphur content in the bulbs which they collected from twelve different parts of Europe. Bulbs gathered near Basel contained only around 500 mg/kg of sulphur, while some from Piacenza in Italy had 1790 mg/kg. Those grown in an experimental garden in Basel had 3720 mg/kg. It may be that these were grown organically. Monsignor David Greenstock, Head of Biology at St Alban's College, Valladolid, in Spain, a world expert on growing and using garlic, found similar variations in bulbs grown in different parts of Spain and noted that they corresponded exactly to the extent to which they were organically grown. Garlic, as one might expect, also does well on sulphur. Feeding sulphur or sulphates dramatically increased its flavor. These variations are significant; size and weight alone are no sure guide to potency, but strength of flavor and amount of sulphur are a guide to potency. It is important to remember this when buying garlic and it will also affect the quality of the various health preparations which contain it.

We have been discussing these essential components in such detail that it may come as a surprise to learn that they make up only a tiny fraction of the bulb. The oil which Semmler extracted weighed between 0.1% and 0.2% of the total, and this is the figure quoted by most experimental scientists. A Mediterranean clove of garlic weighs on average 3 g. while an American-grown garlic clove might weigh 6 g., twice as much. So on that basis there are 3–6 mg. of oil to a small clove and 6–12 mg to a large clove. The alliin/allicin content was generally found to be around 50% higher than the oil content.

Garlic is around 60% water and each clove contains on average 1 g. of carbohydrates (90% of this in a starchy form called sinistrin), 0.2 g. of protein, 0.05 g. fiber, 0.01 g. fat, Vitamin A, Vitamin B1, some Vitamins B2 and B3, and Vitamin C. The thiamine (Vitamin B1) is combined with allicin, something most unusual in the plant world. The combination allithiamine is easily absorbed in the intestine. The Japanese, who first discovered allithiamine, now use it in some of their nutritional supplements.

Another substance in garlic is adenosine, a nucleic acid (a building block of DNA and RNA). As we shall see, it may also contribute to garlic's effects on the blood.

Garlic contains a proportionally high level of trace minerals including copper, iron, zinc, tin, calcium, manganese, aluminium, germanium, and selenium. These last two have attracted the attention of health enthusiasts. Germanium has been discussed as an anti-cancer agent. Selenium, which supports the activity of Vitamins C and E, is present in a concentration of at least 9 p.p.m. It is at a higher level in garlic than any other plant remedy, although it is not important health-wise as we eat such little garlic. The total amount in a clove or two would be much less than in a serving of fish.

Garlic contains about ten different sugars, among them glucose, fructose, arabinose, and inulin. The total sugar content is quite large, amounting to about a quarter of all substances. This confused a key researcher, Runquist, who was working in Scandinavia during World War I. He concluded that the active medical component, which many researchers of the time were looking for, was a sulphur-sugar compound. This view held for some thirty years until it was over-turned by Cavallito and his colleagues. However, it is still propounded in Japan through the work of a Dr. Kominato, who believes that the main medicinal component is a sulphur-sugar with a highly complex structure called scordinin, which is present in rather small amounts—0.03% of the bulb weight. This view must be seen in the light of the Japanese tendency to regard garlic as a restorative nutrient rather than a specific medicine. The Japanese are, on the whole, not so interested in the powerful effects of allicin and diallyl disulphide. Instead, they have looked for odorless constituents which might be nutritious. Despite the general excellence of Japanese natural-product chemists, the weight of evidence is overwhelmingly against scordinin as the active medical ingredient.

There are other substances in garlic which contribute minor themes to the symphony of its taste and smell. Dimethyl disulphide adds a taste of cabbage, propenyl disulphide an onion smell, some isothiocyanates a taste of horseradish and mustard, and some thiophenes a fried onion flavor. When you cut an onion, it is propenyl sulphenic acid which makes you cry.

Because of garlic's importance as a food, its chemistry has been comparatively well researched. The Nobel prize-winner, Professor Artturi Virtanen, together with Dr. B. Granroth and their group of scientists in Helsinki, has analyzed it in such detail that they were able to reveal the interactions of hundreds of different compounds. What we have said here may seem complex, but it is straightforward compared to the total picture. Indeed, all plants contain thousands of constantly changing substances, more than a chemist could ever analyze, and no one could deny that this rich variety also contributes to their value as medicines.

6

Garlic Proved: Against Infections

When we first began looking into the scientific research on garlic, we consulted all the relevant libraries and computer information banks. To our astonishment, we found that some 700 papers had been published over the last twenty years, each one representing a serious investigation. Most of these are studies on isolated tissues or on animals; there are not as many large-scale trials on groups of people as one might wish. Nevertheless their results give impressive scientific backing to the effectiveness of garlic and the wisdom of traditional medicine. One is left marveling at the old doctors, not only because they selected garlic for use but also because they knew so much about it.

In this chapter, we will consider a particular group of uses. Garlic has always had the reputation of being effective against stomach upsets, diarrhea, dysentery, bronchitis, catarrh, throat and ear infections, ulcers, and infected wounds. All these are infections caused by bacteria, harmful bacteria invading the body and overcoming its normal defenses. Other infections, particularly of the skin, are caused by fungi, and garlic was known as a cure for ringworm and for various unpleasant kinds of "scurf." What does the scientific community say about garlic's power against infections? Let us first consider bacteria and begin with one of the great men of science.

Laboratory Culture Studies

In 1858, Louis Pasteur tested the antibacterial properties of both onion and garlic and he found that they killed or stopped the growth of bacteria prepared in culture dishes in his laboratory. At that time garlic was well established as a medicine. Later its use died out, but some researchers on the Continent fought a rear-guard action on its behalf. In 1930, a German scientist, F.A. Lehman, showed that the growth of *Bacillus proteus* bacteria was inhibited by a concentration of garlic extract as low as 1 part in 50,000. Other workers in the 1930s found this effect against staphylococci. Even the blood of people who had eaten garlic killed bacteria. A report in the *Science Weekly* of Frankfurt showed that freshly-crushed garlic could kill bacteria at a distance of twenty centimeters by its vapor alone.

How strong is it, compared to other antibiotics? One paper which deals with this thoroughly appeared in 1977 in the *Indian Journal of Experimental Biology* and came from a team at the University of Pantnagar in India directed by Professor V.D. Sharma. They placed disks of paper soaked in garlic extract in the middle of culture dishes of bacteria and measured the area of the bacteria killed. They found that fresh garlic extract was as capable as any of the common antibiotics to deal with a very wide range of bacteria, including those causing food poisoning, digestive problems, throat, lung, and skin infections, as well as other harmless bacterias. The most effective of the antibiotics tested was chloramphenicol, which worked better than penicillin, tetracycline, streptomycin, and others. Yet garlic matched chloramphenicol and, in two cases, killed bacteria resistant to it.

These kinds of tests have shown that garlic extracts have an unusually broad action against all kinds of bacteria, including bacillus, staphylococcus, escherischia, pseudomonas, streptococcus, vibrio, and mycobacteria species. Garlic, though more indiscriminate than modern antibiotics, is weaker. It is a shotgun, compared to modern antibiotics as marksmen's rifles. Weight for weight, penicillin is fifty times as strong as allicin, and tetracycline is around ten times as strong.

Nevertheless, because it kills all kinds of bacteria, without any harm or toxicity to us, garlic has some great advantages over antibiotics. In particular, where infections keep coming back, or are mild and continuous and never seem to go away, taking garlic may be more effective and safer than repeated doses of antibiotics. Chronic infections of the mouth, gums, throat, ear, chest, stomach, or urinary system are examples. However if the infection becomes acute—with fever, and spreading inflammation—seek medical treatment. Do not expect garlic to deal with it.

Garlic is also very useful to knock out an infection when it first appears. Whenever anyone in Stephen Fulder's family feel the first signs of an infection, such as a sore throat, they immediately have a good course of garlic, together with a raw food diet (mostly fruit), and anti-infective herb teas, particularly sage or thyme. The infection soon goes away. No one in the family has had antibiotics for at least fifteen years.

Another advantage of garlic is that it does not, as far as we know, create bacterial resistance. This occurs when the bacteria get canny: they adapt to the usual antibiotics which become useless. New and often more toxic antibiotics are required. Studies by Dr. Michael Jackson at the University of California at Davis have shown that garlic keeps its power. It can be used repeatedly without risk of bacterial resistance.

How does garlic kill bacteria? It appears that the sulphides in garlic knock out sulphur-containing biological catalysts (enzymes), especially those in and under the coats of the bacteria, which are needed for growth and reproduction. In this, garlic is similar to penicillin, and to its forerunners which were discovered in the 1930s and called sulpha drugs; in all of them it is the sulphur-containing part which does the work.

Let us look at some interesting and well-documented accounts by doctors who used garlic to cure infections.

The Digestive System

Dr. E. E. Marcovici's experiences with garlic began in the trenches of World War I, where he was in charge of experimental studies on preventing and curing gastrointestinal infections. Writing in the *Medical Record* twenty five years later, he described how giving a bulb a day (crushed) to soldiers with dysentery produced a rapid return to health, sometimes within a week. He found some problems with the burning sensations caused in the mouth and stomach, so he made his own ground garlic tablets. Later he used a preparation made by the Sandoz Pharmaceutical Company, in which garlic is combined with charcoal and slowly released as it passes along the digestive tract. After the war, Marcovici conducted experiments to check his wartime experiences. He gave rabbits 2.5 g of garlic powder and found that this completely protected them from a dose of dysenteric organisms ten times the lethal dose.

The bacteria present in the intestines radically change when garlic is eaten. The trouble-makers, for example, those which cause dysentery, enteritis, or "Montezuma's revenge," disappear, and the normal ones return. It is not quite true to say that garlic selects only the unfriendly bacteria for attack. It tends to attack foe rather than friend, but nevertheless knocks out some of each. However, the bacteria which live naturally in the gut soon recover from this, while the invaders do not. Garlic also removes the poisons secreted by some bacteria; one of these is *Escherichia coli*, which sometimes turns ugly and causes stomach upsets. Both Marcovici and Sharma demonstrated that garlic can prevent *E. coli* from making poison. At lower doses, garlic does not kill bacteria but simply stops them multiplying. This gives the body breathing space to marshall its own defenses.

Garlic is also known as a carminative. Like mustard, aniseed, angelica, and fennel, it stimulates the secretion of digestive juices; when the stomach is underactive it encourages it. This was demonstrated in a paper in the *Review of Gastroenterology* by Drs. Damrau and Ferguson, which reviewed twenty-nine successful cures and presented several case reports. For example, a fifty-five year-old woman had, for a year, experienced a whole series of troubles: stomach heaviness and distention after eating, flatulence, continual belching, nervousness, and loss of appetite. She was given two tablets of dehydrated garlic twice daily after meals and, within two weeks, the symptoms were almost gone.

Garlic is the only antibiotic which, at the same time as killing bacteria, also encourages digestion and protects the body against poisons produced by the infection. It may not be as directly lethal to bacteria as some, and may take longer to work. However, its balanced, wide-ranging, and safe action make it an excellent treatment, except in serious cases.

Very recently Professor Mirelman, Professor of Microbiology at the prestigious Weizmann Institute in Israel, has found that garlic extract could kill the amoebas that lead to amoebic dysentery. Fresh garlic extract, or allicin by itself (though not garlic oil) was a powerful amoeba killer that was about one-tenth as potent dose for dose as the leading anti-amoeba drug metronidazole. Professor Mirelman concludes that an allicin-rich garlic remedy could one day benefit millions of entamoeba sufferers throughout the world.

Chest Infections

Garlic is known all over the world as a remedy for chest complaints, especially troublesome and persistent coughs and bronchitis. Laboratory research has been done on this, but there are not many direct studies on patients. However, a few years ago, a Polish group at the Pediatric Institute of the Academy of Medicine in Poznam, under the direction of Dr. T. Ratinsky, studied the effectiveness of garlic treatments on 382 children aged between three months and fifteen years. They obtained their best results with cases of recurrent catarrh and chronic bronchitis. In the USSR and Eastern Europe, garlic is often used today by professional doctors where antibiotics would be prescribed in the West; a certain extract widely sold at Soviet pharmacies has become known as "Soviet penicillin." In 1965, during an influenza epidemic, the *Moscow Evening News* told everyone, "eat more garlic," and the government flew in a 500 metric ton emergency supply.

The use of garlic against tuberculosis has a small chapter of medical history all of its own. At the turn of the century, Dr. William Minchin found himself in charge of the tuberculosis ward of the Kells Union Hospital, Dublin. One day, an eighteen year-old boy with severe tuberculosis of the right leg and foot came to see him, but refused the amputation which Minchin recommended. Six months later he saw the boy in his home town walking without difficulty. It appeared that he had gone to see a farmer, a Mr. Charles Walker of County Meath, who was well known for having a secret remedy for tuberculosis in his family. Minchin discovered that this consisted of a poultice containing soot, salt, and powdered garlic. By experiments, he found the latter to be the active ingredient and from then on used it in his hospital treatments. He applied the oil externally, gave large amounts in the diet and, for tuberculosis of the lung, his patients also inhaled the oil vapors for several hours a day through a specially-made inhaler. He found he could successfully treat almost every case that came to him, provided there was some kind of passage of air to and from the tubercular area; if this was completely shut away, he used surgery. In his book *The Treatment of Tuberculosis with Oleum Allii,* he also recorded the experience of other doctors. Between 1912 and 1914, Dr. M. W. Duffie of the Metropolitan Hospital in New York carried out a large study comparing all known treatments against tuberculosis with 1082 patients. Garlic gave the best results of all. This may be because it permeates the lungs so throughly. Many people have remarked on how quickly and easily it spreads through the body; one doctor even wrote that he could smell it on the breath of babies born to garlic-eating mothers. Tuberculosis is resurfacing, especially in Third World countries, and where modern drugs are not available garlic is an ally. But TB is a serious condition and it is essential to seek medical treatment.

Chest infections on the other hand, which are not so dangerous and far more common, can often be dealt with exclusively by the use of garlic, although the treatment will be much more effective if a therapeutic diet is followed. In fact a new license has been issued for garlic by the Ministry of Health in the United Kingdom which allows manufacturers to claim that garlic is a herbal remedy traditionally used for the treatment of the symptoms of rhinitis and catarrh. Garlic products are more frequently used for these purposes in Northern Europe than for any other reason.

Wounds and Ulcers

Garlic's properties make it a rather effective dressing for wounds, cleansing them and preventing suppuration. It was used for this purpose in front-line dressing stations during World War I. It is said that, in 1916, the British government asked for as much garlic as could be produced and offered a shilling a pound for it, a large price in those days. Penicillin was coming into use during World War II, but supplies were short, particularly on the Eastern front. In 1942, a Russian team of scientists conducted successful experiments on treating war wounds with garlic, and it is known that the Russians used it in the field.

Garlic has traditionally been used in a whole range of external infections. The Poznam study mentioned earlier in this chapter reported very good results in the treatment of children's abscesses. A practicing herbalist described to us the typical case of a man who had a recurrent leg ulcer due to poor peripheral circulation. Garlic cured the ulcer, although the circulation remained defective; he used other plants, like comfrey and aloes, to stimulate the processes of healing and repair. Garlic itself is anti-infective, but will not encourage repair when the infection has gone.

Fungal Infections and Candida

Fungal infections include urethritis, vaginitis, and candida albicans, all of which are caused by a yeast-like fungus of the candida group. There are fungal skin diseases, such as ringworm, tinea, athlete's foot, and certain eye infections, and there are internal infections such as cryptococcosis which is carried by bird droppings and caused by contact with pigeons or chickens.

Fungal infections are rising dramatically in the modern world, in parallel with the decline in bacterial infections—when bacteria go, fungi often take their place. Also many modern treatments, such as the use of steriods and chemotherapy, reduce the effectiveness of the body's immune system, and open the way for fungal infections. Today, candida is a major health problem, causing a wide variety of symptoms, from depression to allergies. The drugs currently used have many disadvantages; they either have an unusually large number of side effects (e.g. amphotericin) or they are not absorbed in the digestion (e.g. nystatin, candicidin). Most of them have to be taken for long periods—typically a month or two as opposed to one or two weeks for bacterial antibiotics—and even after this the infections quite often return.

Research has found that garlic can act as effectively as these agents and more quickly. Drs. Moore and Atkins, at the University of Cambridge in England, found in careful laboratory studies that garlic juice is as strong as the antifungal drugs amphotericin and nystatin. Again it had a much wider range of action, working particularly well against candida, but also against many other kinds of fungi. There are many similar reports from scientists around the world. Candidiasis in farm animals has been successfully treated with garlic. Neal Caporaso and his colleagues at the New Jersey Medical University have even shown that after people took garlic juice, their own blood could kill infecting fungi, although the doses used were high. Because of this kind of research, garlic is now the number one natural treatment for candida infections, in use by thousands of holistic physicians in America.

Other fungal infections, such as that of the skin, are also treatable by garlic. A letter in the *Medical Journal of Australia* of January 23, 1982 from a Dr. Rich of Adelaide recounted how he and all his family were infected with ringworm by a stray kitten. His teenage daughter, the last to suffer, did not think much of the drug the others were using and decided to try garlic instead. Dr. Rich, being a scientific man, persuaded her to treat one arm with garlic and the other with the modern drug; the lesions on her garlic-treated arm healed in ten days, while the other took three to four weeks.

A 1977 study by Robert Fromtling and Glenn Bulmer, of the Department of Microbiology at the University of Oklahoma, on cryptococcosis looked at eighteen different disease-causing strains. They were stimulated by concern about the rise in cryptococcosis—15,000 cases a year in New York alone. They found that all the fungi were killed when small amounts of garlic extract were placed in the dishes where they were growing.

Virus Infections

There are no known drugs of proven use against virus infections. A doctor will prescribe symptomatic treatment—two aspirins and bed rest—for influenza and, for more serious viral infections, like shingles, there are drugs which are only partially effective and toxic, like amantidine. It has often been claimed that garlic helps colds and influenza, and perhaps other viral diseases. If this is true, does garlic work on the infection itself, on the poisons which it produces, or on the body's own immune defenses? Maybe it works because, as traditional medicine would say, it is fiery and induces sweating, which cleanses, cools, and helps the healing process. Dr. Bronwyn Hughes, at Murdock Pharmaceuticals in Utah, in association with colleagues at Brigham Young University, have found clear evidence that garlic or a garlic product, Garlicin, does kill viruses in cells growing in laboratory culture. Some initial evidence indicates that garlic may prevent rather than treat influenza. Science has, as yet, little to offer on the question.

What Works?

What is it in garlic that kills bacteria and fungi? What do the authors of all these studies consider to be the main anti-infective component? Their findings can be summarized as follows:

1. All the studies using garlic juice or fresh garlic found strong effects.
2. Effectiveness decreased with time.
3. If the extracts were boiled, they lost their effectiveness.

The implications of this are clear. The fresh extracts contain allicin, made from alliin, when garlic is crushed. The older extracts had little or no allicin, because it had all changed to diallyl disulphide and other sulphides. In the boiling, some might even have evaporated away. Allicin is therefore the main anti-infection component.

This has been confirmed by a number of researchers, among them Drs. Frank Barone and Michael Tansey at Indiana University. They carefully isolated the component which killed candida and found it to be allicin. They then tested synthetic allicin, which worked well, but was not as strong as the complete fresh extract. So it is likely that there are other unknown anti-infective agents there. However, there is no doubt that allicin is by far the most important one.

Then what about garlic oil—does it work at all against bacteria and fungi? Researchers found that it was less effective than fresh garlic. Pure diallyl disulphide, the main component of the oil, does kill bacteria, but is much weaker than allicin. In one or two scientific studies where a commercial garlic oil capsule was opened and tested on bacteria and fungi, nothing happened. However, it is not known if this is due to the weakness of the oil compared to fresh garlic, or to the small amount of actual garlic oil in the capsule.

Nevertheless, garlic oil capsules have been widely used in Europe for coughs, catarrh, and other infections for at least forty years. One cannot discount the thousands of reports of this kind:

I have suffered from catarrh for years and it was much worse when I moved to my present address. My doctor said that there wasn't really anything he could do and the best thing I could do would be to move to the South of France! A friend recommended garlic pearls, which helped me enormously, but they also benefited me in a way which I was not expecting. I suffer from acne, although I am well past my teens, and to my absolute joy my skin is wonderfully improved.

We are not going to be able to decide on the effectiveness of the oil without clinical studies. Yet it is sure that garlic packs its strongest punch when it is fresh, and rich in allicin.

7

Garlic Proved: In the Circulation

Heart and circulatory disease is now the number one killer in the developed world; just over a half of all deaths are due to it. This chapter, therefore, is perhaps the most vital part of our book. The present-day epidemic has various causes. One is, of course, that deaths from infectious diseases have been greatly reduced, making it possible for more people to die of heart failure. But there is no doubt that our modern way of life, with its lack of physical exercise, its complex worries and tensions, and its various dietary imbalances is creating this kind of disease.

It is now recognized that there should not be too many fats of the wrong sort in the circulation. The dangerous ones are the so-called saturated fats, as well as cholesterol, which are found in high quantities in common foods like meat, dairy products, eggs, lard, and some cooking oils. Drastically reducing the amount of these fats and cholesterol in the diet certainly does reduce the risk of heart problems. But cholesterol is also made by the liver as the body needs some as raw material for the manufacture of hormones. During stressful times the body makes too much. If there is too much cholesterol and fat in the blood it collects on the inside walls of the arteries, which get like old and furred pipes; they become bumpy and ridged and the blood can no longer flow through them smoothly. Arteries get like that from other causes, for example if there are too many stress hormones like adrenaline making their rounds. Unrelieved and nagging stress constricts blood vessels, which raises blood pressure; this also damages the arteries as the blood is forced through more strongly. As the arteries narrow and harden, the heart has to work harder to get the blood around, thereby pushing up the blood pressure; thus there is a vicious circle connecting cause and effect. Less and less oxygen reaches the heart, the most oxygen-hungry organ of the body; lacking oxygen, parts of it die and there is a heart attack.

A further factor plays a part in this and that is the blood's tendency to clot. This stops us bleeding when we cut ourselves but, if the tendency becomes excessive, clots occur internally. The blood builds up clots on the bumps of the artery walls and tiny clots may even begin to circulate, eventually blocking blood vessels and causing thrombosis. This excessive clotting is also related to high fat levels.

Can garlic have an effect on all this and help heart disease? In traditional medicine there are references to it clearing the arteries and purifying the blood. Dioscorides and William Turner make this claim and the *Charaka Samhita* of India says that garlic maintains the fluidity of the blood, strengthens the heart, and prolongs life. Actually, the Ayurvedic traditional medicine of India states that garlic reduces fat in the blood and dries up milk in the breast. Garlic was almost universally recognized as a cure for edema in which poor circulation causes a buildup of water in the tissues. However, circulation problems belong to the modern age; it is from modern research that we get the clearest possible backing for garlic's use.

The Effect on Cholesterol and Other Fats

Work on garlic and the circulation began with Professor Wesselin Petkov in Bulgaria. Petkov was one of the founders of modern research into medicinal plants. He is famous for proving scientifically the old belief that the biological effects of plants vary according to season. In 1949, he artifically induced atherosclerosis (hardening of the arteries) in rabbits by feeding them a diet rich in cholesterol, so that their blood cholesterol levels went sky high. Rabbits that were also given garlic had reduced cholesterol and blood vessels in far better condition. Since then around thirty similar studies have been done. Dr. Bordia and his colleagues at the Rabindranath Tagore Medical College, Udaipur, India, and Dr. Jain at the University of Benghazi, Libya, are the pioneers in this field. In a typical study, cholesterol levels in the blood of the fat-fed animals increased by twenty-five times but in those fed also with garlic only by five times. The blood of the first group showed twice the normal tendency to clot, while with the second, clotting actually became less likely. Studies have also shown that if garlic is given at the same time as fats it reduces the fatty obstructions in the blood vessels by half.

The normal drug given to people at risk of heart disease due to high levels of cholesterol used to be clofibrate. It is still in use, though less so than before. For it was discovered that it actually increased the death rate—from cancer, gall bladder trouble and, ironically, heart attack—of those taking it. *The Lancet* summed it up by saying, "the treatment was successful but unfortunately the patient died." In the studies on fat-fed animals which we have described, garlic was more efficient than clofibrate at lowering cholesterol levels, removing fatty deposits, and reducing the blood's tendency to clot.

Garlic also prevented the animals from becoming obese and had a considerable effect on a blood protein called lipoprotein, which carries cholesterol around the body. It has been shown that where one form of this, HDL (high-density lipoprotein), is present, the heart and arteries are generally healthy and when another form, LDL (low-density lipoprotein), increases, there is more atherosclerosis. Garlic dramatically shifts the balance towards HDL.

Feeding animals extra fat and cholesterol is a rather artificial process and it is perhaps more meaningful to look at the effects of garlic on normally-fed animals. A team of scientists led by Dr. Qureshi at the United States Department of Agriculture laboratories in Madison, Wisconsin, gave a range of doses of garlic extract to chickens, pigs, and other animals, in their normal soya-bean-based diet. Even when garlic formed only 0.2% of their total feed, the chickens were found to have significantly less cholesterol and other fats in their blood.

How Garlic Works

The scientists at Madison, and others at Alcorn State University, Mississippi, and at the famous Wistar Institute in Philadelphia have all investigated how garlic lowers the cholesterol and fats in the body. Quite a clear picture has emerged.

Cholesterol and fat in the blood arrive there from the liver, carried by the LDL (the "unhealthy" lipoprotein). The liver makes its own cholesterol and fat and it also gathers that absorbed in the digestion. Besides this, the liver has a waste-disposal rubbish bag which gets rid of extra fat: the bile gland.

It is now known that garlic acts in two ways. Firstly it increases the dumping of fat and cholesterol by the bile gland. Secondly it actually prevents the liver from making so much fat and cholesterol. It does this because the catalysts which make the fats in the liver rely on sulphur or thiol groups. Garlic's reactive sulphur interferes with these catalysts just as it does that of the bacteria. In this way garlic both prevents loading the liver with fats after a fatty meal, and also lowers the cholesterol in the blood irrespective of the diet.

Enough of animal studies: let us move on to clinical trials with people. The first scientific hint that garlic does the same sort of thing to us was a fascinating study carried out among the Jain community by Dr. Sainani and colleagues of the B.J. Medical Centre in Poona, India. The Jains all share more or less the same vegetarian diet but some, for reasons already described, do not eat garlic or onions, while others do. More than 200 Jains joined the study and were divided into groups similar in age and sex. The first group had a weekly consumption of over 600 g (21 oz) of onion and 50¾g (1 oz) of garlic; the second ate less than 200 g (7 oz) of onion and 10⅓g (oz) of garlic a week, and the third had never eaten either in their lives. They found that the average blood cholesterol levels of the three groups were: group one 159 mg/100 ml; group two 172 mg/100 ml; group three 207 mg/100 ml. These are all levels within the normal range, but they show considerable differences, as did the levels of other fats and of LDL: the more garlic and onion in the diet, the less cholesterol in the blood.

As with the animal studies, it has been quite easy to show that garlic stops the rush of cholesterol in the body straight after a fatty meal. For example Dr. Bordia gave several volunteers a butter-laden breakfast. Their cholesterol levels a few hours later were slightly increased. Where garlic oil was also given with the meal, cholesterol levels were down 10–15%, lower than if they hadn't had any fat. Garlic can take some of the harm out of fatty diets. There is obvious sense in garlic butter, and even more so, in lacing steak with garlic as do the French, who have remarkably low levels of heart disease despite a high fat diet. Mind you, this should be put in perspective—garlic is not, as we shall see, a substitute for taking proper care of yourself. A diet of hamburgers and French fries will be pretty disastrous for your hear in the long run whether or not you eat garlic too.

The real question is, of course, what garlic will do for people with a blood cholesterol problem. Fortunately this question has now been extensively investigated. The pioneering research has come as before, from India. A report published in the *American Journal of Clinical Nutrition* is typical. Twenty healthy volunteers with an average cholesterol level of 233 mg/dl (slightly raised, a level typical for adult male Americans) were given garlic oil equivalent to a head of garlic, each day for six months. The cholesterol levels went down to 200. A comparison group given pretend garlic pills showed no change. When the subjects stopped taking garlic, the cholesterol levels returned. Sixty-two patients who had had a heart attack or heart disease, and who had very high levels of cholesterol, were also given garlic. In this case the cholesterol levels first increased compared to those taking the pretend garlic (placebo), perhaps, as the authors suggest, because fat is being removed from the arteries. Anyway, after some months there was an 18% decrease.

A similar double blind trial has been carried out at the John Bastyr Naturopathic College in Seattle on twenty healthy young people with normal blood cholesterol levels (195 mg/dl). After taking garlic oil for four weeks their blood cholesterol went down to 180 mg/dl. During a similar period in which they took a similar-smelling placebo pill, there was no change in cholesterol.

The major contribution to this work in recent years has come from Germany, where garlic is a licensed medicine for atherosclerosis. Professor Ernst of Munich University started the ball rolling by proving that if patients with high blood cholesterol (260 mg/dl) were put on a diet, their cholesterol fell around 10%. However if dried garlic was added to this diet, the level fell an additional 10%. Garlic seems to go very well with dieting to reduce cardiac risk factors.

Many German scientists jumped on the bandwagon and a string of clinical studies was published, all agreeing that a 10–20% reduction in cholesterol could be expected by using garlic. This culminated in a major study, recently published in the international journal *Drug Research*. It was organized by the German Association of General Practitioners. No less than 261 people who had cholesterol levels over 200 mg/dl, from thirty clinics around Germany, took part. Some were given 800 mg of dried garlic tablets (Kwai brand), equivalent to a small clove of fresh garlic, each day for sixteen weeks. Others were given a placebo. There was a clear 10% reduction in cholesterol in the garlic group along with a 17% reduction in fats, compared to the others.

Some two-thirds of adults in the United States have a somewhat raised blood cholesterol, around 200–250 mg/dl. They are normal healthy people and doctors are reluctant to give them drugs, thereby turning the majority of the U.S. population into patients. A safe, mild, natural remedy like garlic is sorely needed.

The Effect on Blood Clotting

We have already said that garlic has a beneficial effect on the blood's tendency to form clots. Let us now look at this again. Small structures called platelets circulate continuously in the blood. They have a certain "stickiness," that is to say that if they meet any sort of sharp edge or obstruction in the vessels, they adhere to it and begin the complex process of forming a clot. If this tendency increases beyond the normal, webs of a protein called fibrin build up on the walls of the arteries. Tiny clots may also form and circulate dangerously in the blood stream; they cause strokes if they lodge in the vessels of the brain, or coronary thrombosis in those leading to the heart. When it was first proposed that garlic could increase the blood's fibrinolytic or clot-dissolving power, a number of studies were done all over the world to assess the findings. One by Dr. Bordia at Udaipur, on twenty patients who had had heart attacks, showed a 72% increase with one single large dose of garlic and an 80% increase over a month.

Most of the studies on blood cholesterol both in the laboratory with animals, and with people, have also examined the clotting of the blood as it is an easy additional test. In all cases the blood was less sticky and less likely to clot. For example in the John Bastyr College study, blood stickiness dropped by 16% in those taking garlic. A summary of the twenty to thirty studies carried out on garlic and blood stickiness shows that if you take garlic over a period of time, you can expect around a 50% increase in the fibrinolytic, clot-destroying activity of the blood.

The advantage, from a research point of view, of testing garlic's effect on blood clotting is that there is an immediate and very noticeable effect directly after garlic is eaten. By comparison, the effect of garlic on cholesterol builds up slowly over weeks. Studies show that three to four hours after eating fried or raw garlic, the clot-removing activity of the blood increases. Then it gradually falls back to its original level after a day. This indicates that we should take garlic three to four times a day to maintain dose levels in the body.

A study carried out at Saarland University in Saar, West Germany, and published recently in the *British Journal of Clinical Practice*, was done in a unique research lab set up to explore the way the blood flows. It was found that after a subject took garlic powder the blood was more fluid (less viscous). The clot-removing action increased by around 50%. The more garlic taken, the greater the effect.

Besides helping the body to break up clots, garlic also stops the platelets from sticking together and starting the clotting mechanism. This can be confirmed easily by taking a little blood after garlic has been eaten, and checking how long the platelets take to clump. For example in 1981, Dr. David Boullin, working at the Clinical Pharmacology Research Unit at Oxford, UK, tested the blood of people directly after they had eaten garlic. He gave his volunteers four cloves each and found that, an hour afterwards, their blood had lost its ability to stick together; this gradually returned over two and a half hours as the garlic substances were lost or excreted. Dr. Boullin published these discoveries in *The Lancet*. He has done further research which has not yet been published but which he kindly discussed with us. Concerned that his original dose did not realistically reflect people's eating habits, he repeated his experiments using normal dietary amounts, no more than a third of a clove over two daily meals. In order to test this small amount his subects ate no garlic for a month and he then gave them the small garlic doses. He found that their blood was much less sticky after the garlic. In other words only one third a clove a day, the amount anyone can cope with in a normal diet, will prevent thromboses in the blood vessels. The effect is as potent as that of aspirin, which is usually given by doctors in small amounts for this purpose.

How Garlic Stops the Clots

Since the blood stickiness test is so easy to do, it has led to probably the most interesting and sophisticated series of research projects which exists on garlic. Drs. Makheja, Vanderhoek, and Bailey, of George Washington University, Washington DC, took the anti-coagulant properties of garlic and onion seriously. They split garlic oil into various chemical groups, testing each one on blood stickiness. One of these was so effective that, while the normal blood stuck together completely in five minutes, the garlic-treated blood first stuck a little and then returned to a permanently liquid state.

Garlic's sulphur components are again responsible. It seems that they interfere with the enzymes which make prostaglandins. These local messengers are found in platelets, as everywhere else in the body, and they control the way platelets clump. Garlic also reduces the stimulus to clot in the walls of the blood vessels themselves. It does so by restricting the catalysts which make thromboxane (which promotes clotting) and encouraging the opposite, prostacyclin, which delays clotting. Aspirin works in a somewhat similar way.

You may feel that it would be unwise to thin the blood and delay the clotting process. In fact, in the modern world most people's blood clots too easily. It goes with cholesterol and fats; if these are excessive, clotting is faster. Garlic brings it back to normal. Large quantities of garlic can be consumed without any danger of excessive bleeding. Nevertheless it would be wise to check with a doctor about taking garlic along with anti-coagulant drugs, and not to take garlic just before surgery.

High Blood Pressure

Cholesterol levels are a rather recent story. Previously, people used to worry most about their blood pressure as a sign of how their heart was doing. Garlic used to be taken against high blood pressure, and until very recently, this was the main East and Central European use of it. There are many pre-war East European scientific reports showing that garlic can reduce the blood pressure of animals, as well as patients with high blood pressure or hypertension. It was thought at the time that garlic worked by cleaning up the intestine, thereby removing poisons that raised blood pressure.

A typical study was carried out in 1966 by garlic's pioneer researcher, Professor Petkov. On giving garlic to 114 hypertensive patients he found a 20–30 mm/Hg drop in systolic pressure and a 10–20 mm/Hg drop in diastolic pressure. Such a change could tip the scale from dangerous to safe. On the other hand many of the early studies on blood pressure were somewhat unreliable. We now know that many things can affect blood pressure—even attention from doctors or nurses can bring it down—so it must be studied carefully.

Recent research has tended to partly confirm these early reports. Garlic does lower raised blood pressure, but it is a mild drop, and the blood pressure raises again afterward. Dr. Foushee and colleagues at North Carolina Central University, Durham, found that when high doses of garlic juice were given to rats with chronic high blood pressure, the blood pressure dropped to normal, at least for twenty-four hours.

Several modern clinical trials using placebos and double-blind methods have been completed in Europe between 1988 and 1990. Small doses of dried garlic powder were used, and it was found that those subjects with high blood pressure experienced a drop of 5–10% over several weeks.

A German study compared twenty hypertension pa-

tients given garlic pills with the same number given reserpine, a standard blood pressure lowering drug. Neither
the patients nor their doctors knew which was which.
Garlic dropped the blood pressure from 176 over 99 to
164 over 85, a modest drop of around 7%. Reserpine
was slightly more effective.

The drop in blood pressure is more likely due to garlic's
known effects on prostaglandins than to any effect on the
intestines. For prostaglandins control the tightening and
loosening of blood vessels. The fine blood vessels on the
outside of the body expand slightly after garlic is taken.
Some ingenious experiments have proved this by mea-
suring, with delicate instruments, the easiest blood vessels
to see: those at the back of the eyes.

Garlic is not a specific medicine for high blood pressure. There are other herbs that are more effective.
Nevertheless its effects on blood pressure are most useful
as a complement to those on fat and cholesterol. Indeed
it is the only remedy known to help both raised fats and
raised blood pressure. Garlic is ideal for lifelong prevention and protection of the heart and circulation. It is also
a total medicine for those who have mild atherosclerosis.
Instead of taking a pill to deal with cholesterol, another
to lower blood pressure, another as a diuretic, and aspirin
against clotting, each with its side effects, it can be done
all at once, safely, with garlic. And it may even make that
cardiovascular diet less of a punishment.

The Effect on Blood Sugar

It has been known for a long time that garlic lowers the
sugar level in the blood. Central and Eastern European

folk medicine used it regularly for this purpose. Of course the herbalists of history knew nothing of blood sugar levels. But they would have noticed the debility that results from mild diabetes and would have used garlic as a "tonic."

Several studies confirm that garlic does reduce blood sugar levels, at least in animals. The effect is mild, and in this case garlic's cousin, the onion, scores more points. For example a study was done on animals by Drs. Chang and Johnson at the United States Department of Agriculture Laboratories in Beltsville, Maryland, to determine whether the liver changes the way it handles fats and sugars when garlic is eaten. Using radioactive "labels" on fats and sugar in the body, they found that fat manufacture in the liver went down by half. Blood sugar also went down, as the liver took sugar out of the blood to store it. The reason was that more of the hormone insulin was released into the bloodstream. How garlic encourages the pancreas to release insulin is, at present, unknown.

This has not been proved in studies with people so one should be cautious about recommending garlic in this case. However it would be fair to say that garlic, along with a diet, could be helpful to those with high blood sugar, and there is no harm in trying it along with other treatments.

What Works on the Circulation?

It is the fresh, allicin-containing garlic which has the most anti-infective properties. For thinning the blood, however, the fresh and the older or heated oil extracts work equally well. This is also true for the anti-cholesterol properties, for researchers fried and boiled their cut garlic or used garlic oil and found it just as good at reducing fats. The same holds true for the effect on blood pressure.

So any kind of garlic will protect the circulation, provided it contains those odorful sulphur ingredients. Moreover, to check which ones are the most potent, garlic is broken down into its components and the active ones are individually tested to determine their blood-thinning properties. Within one hour after these garlic compounds are taken it is possible to check the stickiness of the blood.

This has been done by several researchers, including the teams at George Washington University and New York State University, as well as others in the Department of Chemistry at the University of Delaware and the College of Medicine of the University of Utah. The results are interesting. Ajoene was discovered by Eric Block to be a powerful anticlotting compound. It astonished many scientists when it was described in a major article in *Scientific American*. Though it is not present in fresh garlic or garlic products, it is being investigated as a possible new anti-coagulant drug. In fresh garlic it is allicin which has blood-thinning properties, while in the oil there are several compounds with as powerful effects as allicin. One, discovered in Japan, is methyl ally trisulphide (MATS) which makes up about 5% of garlic oil. Another compound which the George Washington University team felt to be the main one in the oil is called dimethyl trisulphide, or DITS as we might christen it. They also found that adenosine, present in small quantities in fresh garlic is extraordinarily rich, is highly active against blood clotting. Each of the above compounds is potent. The effect of whole garlic or its products will thus be the sum of all its active components.

In Conclusion

Garlic researchers at a United States Department of Agriculture laboratory ended their work when they found that rats' blood smelled of garlic. Said one, "It just doesn't seem to me that anyone would be interested in smelling that much of garlic, no matter what it could do for them." Alas for White Anglo-Saxon Protestants! Our distaste may be giving us dis-ease!

Why is it that heart disease is highest in garlic hating countries and lowest in garlic eating ones? For example, it is a well-documented fact that the Mediterranean peoples have less heart trouble than those of Northern Europe despite eating a great deal of meat. There was recently a discussion of this question in *The Lancet*. One doctor wrote saying it was because, statistically, they ate more garlic; another wrote to say that they drank more wine; yet another that they ate less fat but that there were so many factors it was impossible to be certain about any of them. However, one can carry logic-chopping too far; the overall picture is clear. Don't eat without allium; don't cook without a clove.

Nowadays, we are given a great deal of advice on how to keep our hearts and circulation healthy. We should exercise to keep fit. We are told to eat less saturated fats, meat, salt, caffeine, and sugar and to avoid worry and stress. Then there is magnesium, vitamin E, B vitamins, GLA, fish oil, and a host of useful herbs. All these help, yet sometimes one is confronted with so many suggestions that it is difficult to know where to start and difficult to put them all into practice. Garlic has much to offer because it works on so many of the factors connected with the heart and circulation. It does not, let us be clear, improve the functioning of the heart. However, it can help in many other ways, lowering cholesterol and fat levels, reducing clotting, lowering blood pressure, removing toxins, and encouraging the elimination of excess salt and water. Garlic is the perfectly balanced preventive remedy for the circulation. There could be no better first step than taking it.

8
Garlic Purifier

Infa e' thoum was a Cairo street-sellers' cry—garlic is useful. In this chapter, we will discuss what we consider to be garlic's remaining uses and whether they can be confirmed by science. Many, though not all, of these have to do with its ability to combat poisons.

Bites and Stings

In the past, one of garlic's most popular virtues was as an antidote to poisonous bites and stings. Almost every herbalist mentions "venomous beasts" of some kind: snakes, scorpions, spiders, shrew-mice, toads, dogs, mad and otherwise, and even the bites of men. Nowadays, we have more powerful and specific anti-toxins for dangerous snake bites and for rabies. But there are toxic bites, for example from scorpions, which are painful and for which antidotes are not used. Country people, such as the Druze villagers, often put garlic on these bites. Stephen Fulder and his family also use it when they are unlucky enough to get a scorpion bite, and it is effective. Speed is of the essence; you must cut a clove and rub it on the bite before the poison begins to spread. Garlic may neutralize the toxins by means of its sulphur components. Bites from insects such as fleas and mosquitoes are not helped by garlic, since the pain they cause is almost entirely due to inflammation. Nor will it help with bee or wasp stings.

Garlic has the reputation of discouraging all kinds of biting creatures. Indian women put it in the oil they rub on their hair and it keeps off head lice. Farmers in many parts of the world have found that it helps keep their animals free of ticks and a modern Russian scientific study confirmed this. Vampires and vampire bats may be different sorts of phenomena, but garlic repels both. In Central and South America, where the bats live, it is said that they will not attack horses which have been fed on it. (Incidentally, vampire bats secrete an anti-coagulant in their saliva which keeps the blood of their victims flowing smoothly. Science does not reveal the anti-coagulant employed by Count Dracula.)

Worms and Parasites

Garlic was frequently used in the past to expel intestinal worms. One can well understand how any worm living comfortably in the gut would be repelled by garlic's sulphurous fumes. The thread worms or pinworms that live inside the anus are especially sensitive to it. If garlic is taken by children with pinworms, large numbers are passed out, inert. Scientific evidence for this is scanty; few researchers have shown interest in exploring this less dramatic territory. However, in poorer countries the problem of internal parasites is truly enormous. As you read this eight billion roundworms are sheltering in intestines around the world. Garlic's ancient reputation should be urgently tested.

Metal Poisoning

Let us now consider poisons of a more typically modern sort. Minerals in the body are usually held in place by sulphur compounds. Since these can capture atoms of metals it is to be expected that garlic's sulphur can catch and remove unwanted toxic metals.

Professor Kitahara of Tokyo has indeed shown that garlic juice will trap a tenth of its own weight of lead or mercury, which are highly toxic. Professor Petkov showed that garlic can reduce the signs of chronic lead poisoning in industrial workers; over a hundred took the Bulgarian garlic preparation Satal and blood indications of heavy metal contamination were considerably reduced. In Japan, a growing awareness of industrial pollution led to some unique studies on how a garlic preparation can help remove toxins. When mercury was fed to rats, those given the preparation eliminated it two to three times faster. In the test tube, the garlic extract directly protected blood cells from the destructive effects of heavy metals, and there is evidence that it works by helping the liver neutralize poisons.

It is an exciting possibility that what we eat can help neutralize some of the many contaminants and pollutants in our bodies. A campaign for a clean environment should also include our inner environment and, so far, medical science has not seriously investigated this subject.

Poisons from Bacteria and Fungi

We said in chapter six that, when dealing with infections, garlic also neutralizes the poisons given off by bacteria and fungi. Dr. Marcovici, for example, described how it counteracted the toxins from the dysentery-causing organism, shigella. If this is true, it is striking, for modern pharmacology has failed to come up with drugs to block these often unpleasant by-products. Diseases caused by eating food contaminated by fungi are extremely common, especially in Third World countries. Aflatoxin, for example, is an extremely potent poison, sometimes occurring in moldy peanuts. Monsignor David Greenstock, writing in *Ceres,* a Spanish language agricultural journal, has made a strong case that garlic is perhaps the only material which is capable of counteracting such poisons.

Hangovers

While on the subject of poisons, we should not forget the friendliest and most often welcomed. "Garlic, in strongly exciting the digestion, quickly dissipates drunkenness," says a nineteenth-century paper on the subject. Garlic is widely used on the Continent "the day after;" there is a special garlic and onion soup known as *soupe a l'ivroigne.* In fact, the hangover problem is largely due not to alcohol but to other more toxic substances, such as aldehydes, also produced in the fermentation process. Garlic, by its heating, diuretic, and anti-toxic properties is likely to be of help but to our knowledge this has never been seriously studied. It is worthy of formal (and informal) experiment.

Oxidation

If fruit goes brown or fat turns rancid, it is simply gathering oxygen from the air. Vitamin C halts this process, as do Vitamin E, selenium, and linked sulphur amino acids, like glutathione. The latter two are found in garlic, which is known to be an efficient anti-oxidant. Nowadays food preservatives are either anti-bacterial or anti-oxidant, but garlic meets both requirements. It is, in fact, quite often used as a preservative and has been since earliest times, especially by nomadic herdsmen. There are several scientific papers on the subject, including one on the preservation of camel meat!

Cancer

It is difficult to distinguish treatments for cancer in the old herbals, but Pliny, the *Anglo Saxon Leech Book,* and the medieval herbalist, Macer, speak of applying garlic in fat or lard to tumors or swellings. We have met people who believe that taking large quantities of garlic can treat cancer, a practice which comes from German folk medicine. There has been some very interesting scientific work on this. Significant studies began with Dr. Weisberger, of Case Western University in Cleveland, Ohio. He was fascinated by the antibacterial properties of garlic. He knew they were the result of its interference with the thiol groups which bacteria need for their growth, and particularly for cell division. Perhaps the growth of cancer cells which, like bacteria, divide more quickly than normal cells could be similarly halted? In 1953, Weisberger and his colleague, Pensky, mixed cancer cells with small quantities of allicin and then injected them into mice. These mice were still alive six months later while those without allicin died within sixteen days.

This led to further studies. A researcher in Germany demonstrated that garlic can cause the regression of certain tumors, particularly breast tumors in mice, but other cancers, such as leukemia, were unaffected. In Japan, the researchers Kamura and Yamamoto, at the University of Hokkaido (where the best Japanese garlic grows), confirmed that garlic extracts prevented the divison of cancer cells growing in the human body. They agreed with Weisberger; it seemed as if the thiol groups were responsible.

All this is interesting, but in no way conclusive enough to support claims that garlic can cure cancer. Much more research is needed and, fortunately, it seems that more is on the way. In 1982, Dr W. E. Criss and his team at Howard University, Washington DC, showed that injected garlic extract slowed the growth of liver cancers in animals by 50%. There was evidence that it was blocking the action of an essential growth enzyme. In 1983, Sidney Belman, of the New York University Medical Center, published a paper showing that garlic protected the body from cells that were on their way to becoming cancerous and concluded that having garlic in one's diet could be a useful preventitive.

This has been confirmed by Dr. Michael Wargovitch at the University of Texas System Cancer Center, who published a report that attracted media attention worldwide. He demonstrated that garlic, especially the sulphide groups in garlic oil, helps the liver to destroy cancer-causing chemicals, and thus prevents cancer. Put another way, if your food is full of additives and pesticides, at least lace it with garlic too!

Evidence of a general nature in support of this comes from China. Dr. Mei Xing of Shandong Medical College found that Gangshan county in that province had a very low death rate from stomach cancer; the county next door, Qixia, had a rate more than ten times higher. Their diets were similar, apart from the fact that the people of Gangshan regularly ate up to 20 g, that is to say nearly a whole head of garlic, a day, while their neighbors hardly ate any.

Some reports have suggested that germanium, which is present in garlic in comparatively large amounts, can prevent and cure cancer. This is an interesting possibility but it has not yet been proved and Weisberger's ideas on garlic's effects seem more plausible. We must hope that scientists continue to take its potential as a cancer preventive seriously.

Garlic's Side Effects

Garlic removes poisons; can it be a poisoner? Hippocrates wrote, "garlic causes flatulence, a feeling of warmth in the chest, and a heavy sensation in the head; it excites anxiety and increases any pain which may be present." "In the group to which raw garlic (5 g/kg body weight) was administered, five rats died of the serious stomach injury in twenty-one days," wrote more modern investigators from Japan. These sources both refer to the side effects of garlic. We would expect it to have some; any medicinal agent which has one desired effect on the body will also have other "side" effects. But what are these and how undesirable are they?

There is no doubt that fresh garlic irritates; eating it causes a burning sensation in the mouth and perhaps the stomach as well. To moderate this, it should always be taken with at least some water. The effect is temporary and passes away; it is caused by allicin, and garlic oil creates no such discomfort. However, if the contact with fresh garlic is prolonged, for example if it is repeatedly placed in the gums or on wounds, then blistering can occur. In fact, it was used in this way to draw out poisons by means of an artificial inflammation—hence its description as a rubefacient. The effect on the stomach only becomes serious at impossibly high doses. The rats which died were given five grams of fresh juice per kilogram body weight, the equivalent of 350 grams for a seventy kilogram man; this is like eating at least one kilogram of garlic or 300 perfectly mashed cloves at one sitting! Even then, many of the rats completely recovered from this massive dose. In some studies, the equivalent of twenty cloves was given to people daily for three months without any signs of ill effects, besides the passing burning sensations. There have been studies in which people were given 200 mg of oil, the equivalent of seventy cloves per day, with no signs of side effects. Garlic emerges with a clean bill of health from the standard laboratory safety tests, including those on the causing of cancer.

A concerted effort has been made by Japanese interests to demonstrate that normal garlic is toxic. The paper which showed rats killed by huge doses is quoted as proof of the particular harmfulness of allicin, and is part of an attempt to market deodorized garlic preparations which do not contain allicin or diallyl disulphide. The marketing strategy is to depict allicin as an enemy rather than a friend. We would beg to differ.

For certain people, however, undesirable side effects can occur and we should be aware of them. Some people who are particularly sensitive to foods can be allergic to garlic and suffer from rashes, flushes, asthma, or headaches. If they handle garlic they may break out in skin rashes. It is probably the sulphur compounds which are responsible, since studies have shown that the allergy-causing materials are soluble in water and destroyed by heating or cooking. Allergic reactions are, thankfully, rare but they should be watched for by sensitive individuals. Onions and garlic cause more skin reactions than any other vegetables.

There are other people who, while not being allergic to garlic, still find it difficult to take. They may experience nausea, stomach upsets, thirst and dryness, or headaches. These are often transient and may even indicate that it is having a remedial effect. Garlic is, nevertheless, pungent stuff; if you have such reactions you should reduce your consumption or mix the garlic with other carminatives, like fennel, dill, or caraway.

9

Garlic Pesticide

The plant world breeds many natural defenders of its own kingdom. There is pyrethrum from *Chrysanthemum cinerariaefolium* and there is the Indian neem tree, which has recently provided several pesticides. Garlic, likewise, has the killing of pests among its many powers. Growing it near other plants keeps them free of aphids, or so gardeners all over the world say. Some put it near their roses, others put cloves at the corners of their orchards or line the borders of their vegetable beds with garlic soldiers and believe that pests will be less willing to pass.

The most vocal promoter of the use of garlic as pesticide is Monsignor David Greenstock, whom we have already mentioned. He first tried to control attacks by the onion fly, which does so much damage in his part of Spain. He tried planting garlic around the outside of his onion beds but this did not work. Then he tried growing alternate lines of garlic and onions and found that the onions were almost completely protected. He found dead larvae around the onion bulbs and reasoned that garlic gave off a secretion through its roots which killed them.

Greenstock continued his work by trying to find a garlic solution which would be an effective pesticide. Like so many researchers, he worked by trial and error. First he tried boiling garlic in water, but this did not work. Then he tried a 5% emulsion made from garlic oil and this gave excellent results. In the laboratory, almost every one of the insects and their larvae died. In the field, it was harder to estimate success because, when the insects got a whiff of the garlic, they bolted. He used garlic with success on wireworm, cockchafer larvae, mole crickets, grey field slugs, cabbage-white and ermine-moth caterpillars, and pea weavils. In the end, he found it ineffective against Colorado beetles but this also meant that, unlike other pesticides, it did not harm similarly-sized friendly creatures, such as ladybirds. His home recipe for an insecticide has appeared in several books and journals and has killed many pests. One of the authors of this book has used it successfully against blackfly and used it regularly as a preventive wash in his organic vegetable garden. Here it is:

Soak thirty minced cloves of garlic in 2 teaspoonsful (10 ml) of mineral oil (e.g. paraffin) for 24 hours. Dissolve 7 g ($^1/_4$ oz) of an oil-based soap in 600 ml (1 pt) of water and add it to the garlic, stirring thoroughly. Strain and store the liquid in a glass or ceramic container. Use it as a spray on your plants at a dilution of between 1 part in 20 and 1 part in 100 of water. (Take the dilutions seriously because if it is too strong, it can burn your plants.)

Other cultivators are less exact in the way they make their insecticide. They take crushed whole bulbs, skins or remains of plants, put them in a tub with water, and leave it all to stew. The insecticidal components of garlic are the oil sulphides which last for some time. After a few weeks or months they will decay but, as long as the mixture is primed with fresh material, there is no reason why it should not work.

Garlic's ability to kill insects was backed up by a scientific study by S.V. Amonkar and E.L. Reeves, made in 1969 at the University of California. They had noticed that a certain kind of algae, which is toxic to mosquito larvae in water, gave off a garlicky smell. They made up two solutions, a simple dilution of a garlic extract and another of garlic oil. They tested these at different concentrations on various species of mosquito larvae, including one that was highly resistant to pesticides. With the first extract, all the larvae died at dilutions of between 100 and 200 p.p.m. (or one garlic clove in 15 liters (4 gal) of water). With the second, they died at between 30 and 50 p.p.m. Amonkar subsequently showed that oil of fresh garlic was even stronger; it killed all the larvae at 1 teaspoonful (5 ml) of garlic juice in 1000 l (264 gal). He also demonstrated that the active ingredients were diallyl disulphide and diallyl trisulphide.

If garlic can kill parasites and fungi in human beings and animals, it ought to do the same for plants. In fact, garlic has been found to be a very useful garden fungicide. Farmers used to spray it on grapes in Spain to control wilt or yellowing of the leaves.

Another useful procedure is to put a garlic clove into the hole before planting a cabbage, cauliflower, or other vegetable of the *Cruciferae* family: this keeps them from getting club root. This was proved to be effective in experiments at the Good Gardener's Association. Club root is a most persistent fungus infection, malforming roots and rotting them from the inside.

Scientific studies have also been made of garlic as a fungicide. Peter Ark, Professor of Plant Pathology at the University of California in Berkeley, showed that spraying with a 1% solution of garlic-water extract and dusting with dried garlic powder stopped downy mildew of cucumber and radish, bean rust, anthracnose, brown rot of fruit, and blight of tomatoes and beans. Another good tip emerges from this: before storing your apples for the winter, dip them in a garlic solution.

A study at the Department of Plant Sciences of Indiana University at Bloomington, Indiana, compared the amount of bacteria and fungi in soils in which garlic is grown to soils which had been garlic-free for several years. Indeed, the garlic soils had much less bacteria than the other soils although there was not much difference in the amount of fungi. The kinds of bacteria and fungi in the soil were also changed.

Garlic's great advantage is that it is completely harmless to its users and to birds and animals. It is weaker than pesticides when applied in nature, so it needs to be given more often. However today there are few safe pesticides and fungicides. There must be many people saying to themselves, "I don't like putting poisons on my plants; find me something safer and I'll use it." To such people we say, "try garlic."

10

Garlic Products

Fresh Garlic

Freshly crushed garlic is undoubtedly the strongest form. It has all the allicin in the original clove, and none of it will have started down the slippery slope of chemical changes. Yet fresh garlic has a powerful smell, and the allicin is pungent and burning. How can we reduce this? When garlic is chewed, most of the odor is from leftovers in the mouth. The rest is from the stomach, and after some time there is a little odor from the lungs and skin. The mouth odor can be prevented by swallowing crushed garlic with water, soup, or milk, and other odors reduced by "chasing" the garlic with parsley, cress, or aromatic seeds such as aniseed and fennel. More of this in the next chapter.

You can try some creative ways to take garlic. One day a visitor to Stephen Fulder's farmhouse saw what to her was an amazing sight. There in the kitchen sat his six-year-old daughter who with great concentration and a serious expression was inserting slivers of peeled cloves into grapes. "What on earth are you doing?" said the visitor. "I'm preparing my medicine," she answered, and forthwith popped one after another into her mouth.

Freshly crushed garlic in food will work as a medicine, but you must make sure that you consume a sufficient dose as some of the medicinal value is lost with this method. Also, don't forget that heating will destroy the allicin.

Yet fresh garlic is a bit much for most people, especially if they are not used to it in their diet. Fortunately there are a wide range of products available which reduce or eliminate the odor and the pungency of fresh garlic. As one might expect, they are extremely popular in countries where garlic is not often used in cooking. Today garlic tablets are among the best-selling of all remedies in German pharmacies. In Europe as a whole they are the top selling over-the-counter remedy for circulatory problems. Three-hundred million capsules a year are sold in the United Kingdom. Around $100 million worth of garlic products are sold in the United States every year.

But this very popularity has brought a great deal of confusion to consumers. Every manufacturer claims his product is the best, often deluging shopkeepers and members of the public with conflicting quasi-scientific data. You would need a Ph.D. to work through this material, and even then you wouldn't know who to believe. So let us look at the different ways garlic is made into products and the strengths and weaknesses of each type.

Garlic Oil Capsules

These were the first of all garlic products. Originally called garlic pearls, they were devised in Europe in the

1920s and are still popular there, and especially in the United Kingdom. Garlic oil is usually made by distillation. Steam is bubbled through a mash of crushed garlic, from which the essential oil of garlic is condensed. The oil contains only the oily sulphides made when allicin breaks down, and is roughly equivalent to crushed fried garlic.

The oil is the strongest smelling of all garlic products. However after distillation it is diluted with vegetable oil and put into one-piece capsules. When swallowed whole, they pass straight into the stomach, before dissolving, thus avoiding almost all the taste and smell. The smell is sometimes further controlled by coating the capsule with an "enteric" coating which delays the release of its contents until it has passed through the stomach, into the intestine.

Garlic oil capsules are much less effective than fresh garlic against infections, as we have already discussed. However they are fully active in protecting the circulation. They are also an inexpensive form of taking garlic.

The problem with oil capsules is that they very often contain very small amounts. Let us consider the quantities involved. Garlic oil is extremely concentrated. Semmler and other chemists found that, when they distilled garlic, they produced between 1 and 2 g of oil for every kilo of garlic. This means that the oil is 0.1–0.2% of the total content. This is very similar to the figure of 0.1–0.3% given in the definitive pharmaceutical handbook, *Martindale's Extra Pharmacopoeia*. Now if we say that a small clove weighs 3 g, it will have 3 to 6 mg of oil. Garlic oil capsules generally contain around 0.7 mg of oil, which means that you would need to take 5 to 10 of them to obtain the equivalent of one small garlic clove.

The weakness of the commercial oil capsules has been confirmed on more than one occasion where clinical studies which used them failed to confirm cholesterol lowering and other effects. Laboratory-made garlic oil worked, commercial capsules did not. As one clinical researcher, Dr. R.R. Sampson of the Royal Infirmary in Edinburgh, wrote, "our findings indicate that the garlic content in proprietary health food capsules is insufficient to alter platelet aggregation." So if you take garlic oil capsules, take many.

Dried Garlic Products

These are a newer and more modern way of preparing medicinal garlic products. They have the advantage that they contain whole garlic in a dry form, so more of the constituents may be present. There are two main types of dried garlic products. Since both of them aim to release both allicin and sulphides in the intestine, the dried garlic products should be effective for all garlic's uses. Dried garlic powder is also much easier to analyse chemically than the oil. Companies making the powder products have packets a reasonable level of allicin. This is a great plus for these dried garlic products. For if a herb has a defined level of active substances, it added to a growing list of herbs, from ginseng to gingko that have been standardised. It is an end to the old uncertainties about the dosages and effectiveness of plant remedies, and ushers in the age of hebal "phytopharmaceuticals."

The alert reader will notice something contradictory in the above paragraph. It is this. How can allicin levels be guaranteed in a product if allicin is unstable and spontaneously changes to its sulphide daughter substances. This is indeed a good question and the answer is this: that the garlic powder products do not actually *contain* allicin. They mostly contain the precursors, alliin and allinase, which make allicin on dissolving in water or in the juices of the intestine. So it would be more correct to say that the products guarantee not allicin itself but "allicin yield." Since they contain mostly the precursors, alliin and enzyme, they are also relatively odorless, the odour being released only when the powder is dissovled in liquid inside the body. This is the third advantage of this kind of product.

Such products are made in two basic ways.

1. Odor-Controlled Powder Capsules

One way to remove most of the odor from garlic without losing its activity is as follows. Garlic is first treated to stop the conversion of alliin to allicin. Then it is crushed and dried. This results in a powder which contains the alliin of the original clove but no allicin. Allinase is added to the powder and it is put into hard capsules. Allicin is made only when the capsule is dissolved or digested. The active odorful ingredients are released only after the capsule is swallowed. The advantage of this method is that the capsules contain 100% garlic powder without the need for any oils or diluents. The disadvantage is that no one knows how much allicin is actually made after digestion.

2. Partially Odorful Tablets and Capsules

There are other ways to reduce odor and make a garlic powder that releases allicin on digestion. These mostly involve manipulating the way in which garlic is cut and sliced and the conditions under which it is dried. Garlicin is a product of this type. Kwai Garlic is another one; it is made in the following way. Garlic slices are dried and ground. The powder is made into small tablets which are also enteric coated. The powder thus contains some of the sulphides (where the garlic is cut) plus uncombined alliin and allinase (from inside the slices), which, again, combine after swallowing to make allicin.

Aged Odorless Garlic Extracts

Aged odorless garlic extracts are made by chopping garlic and aging it in alchohol over a long period. It is then extracted, and prepared as a liquid product, or dried and made into tablets or capsules. Aged extracts, which originated in Japan, do not appear to have garlic's main medicinally active ingredients, such as allicin or diallyl disulphide. Indeed, Japanese producers have stated that allicin is harmful and the aged product is advantageous in not having any. However this is contrary to a tremendous amount of scientific and clinical work over the last fifty years which is unequivocal: garlic's main active ingredients are the odorful ones.

This raises serious doubts about the medicinal activity of this type of preparation. "Totally odorless garlic preparations are ineffective" writes one scientist in the prestigious publication *The Lancet* of 15 January 1990. Of course such odorless preparations may have nutritional value or may be active in some peripheral uses of garlic, such as anti-toxicity, for which the active compounds are not yet established.

Garlic Food Products

There are also many kinds of garlic products sold as food, such as garlic paste, or powdered or granular dried garlic. In principle these products will contain the ingredients you expect to find in garlic. However as they are often dried with heat and are not fresh, they will not contain allicin, and the longer they have been stored the less effect they will have, as the sulphides slowly disappear. They may have similar medicinal properties to the oil capsules, but their effects will be unreliable. Furthermore they have the same smell as fresh garlic without the medicinal benefit. So it is preferable to take fresh garlic or capsules or tablets rather than garlic food products.

We can briefly summarize the nature of the various garlic products in Figure 4, which compares how they are made, and the results. It is fair to say that dry powder garlic products are preferable to garlic oil capsules at their usual dosage because of the small amount of oil in the capsules. It is not possible to decide on the relative effectiveness of the various kinds of powder garlic products without comparative studies. However, you should compare how much garlic there is in the products and look for standardization: guaranteed potency. It is worth remembering that all garlic products are effective if their dissolved contents smell and taste strongly of garlic. If you are not sure, open a capsule or tablet and try it.

Figure 4: Garlic Products: How are they made? What is inside?

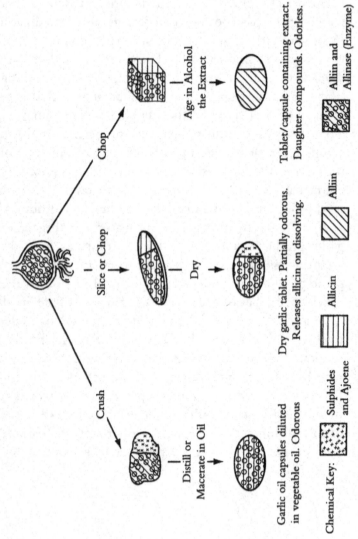

Crush → Distill or Macerate in Oil

Garlic oil capsules diluted in vegetable oil. Odorous

Slice or Chop → Dry

Dry garlic tablet. Partially odorous. Releases allicin on dissolving.

Chop → Age in Alcohol the Extract

Tablet/capsule containing extract. Daughter compounds. Odorless.

Chemical Key:

Sulphides and Ajoene

Allicin

Alliin

Alliin and Allinase (Enzyme)

11

Garlic Preparations

In this chapter, we will present some practical conclusions based on research, both ancient and modern. The table on page 103 shows conditions for which we consider garlic can be used as all or part of the treatment. In the first column, under "general use," are the health problems which, according to all the evidence, can be helped by garlic. The second column, that of "limited use," indicates where it *may* be of help.

Dosages

What is the right amount of garlic to take? Recommended dosages of garlic vary considerably. The early herbals contained no precise amounts, either because they were a matter of common custom or because they were left to the individual art of the herbalist. However, one can often infer the sort of quantities involved. These days, one finds enormous variations in recommended doses, from the gigantic to infinitesimal. Deciding on

Medicinal Uses for Garlic Preparations

Part of body	General Use	Limited Use
Chest and head	Bronchitis Catarrh Laryngitis Sore throats Tonsillitis	Colds Coughs Middle-ear infections Sinusitis
Mouth	Gum infections Mouth ulcers	
Digestive system	Diarrhea Dysentery Food poisoning Indigestion	Gastroenteritis Colitis Constipation Hemorrhoids
Urogenital	Candidiasis Cystitis Thrush Vaginitis	
Skin	Absesses Athlete's foot Yeast-like infections	Acne Ringworm Suppurating wounds Ulcers

Circulation and metabolism	Atherosclerosis
	High blood cholesterol
	High blood fat
	Tendency to vascular
	  thrombosis
		High blood
		  pressure
		High blood
		  sugar

Others	Poisoning from heavy
	  metals and some
	  other contaminants
	Bacterial and fungal toxins
	General nutritional tonic
	Threadworms
	Bites(non-lethal)
		Bee stings
		Debility
		Hangovers
		Lice and ticks
		Round worms
		Skin and hair
		  tonic

what is suitable is far from straightforward. When one considers that the soil in which the garlic is grown, the methods and especially the temperatures used in preparing extracts, their age and how they are stored, all will affect potency, and that different kinds of extracts are suitable for different purposes, one can get an idea of the complexity involved—a complexity never thoroughly investigated. We will attempt to be as precise as we can by describing three levels of dosage. (Please note: all metric conversions in this chapter are approximate.)

Very High, "Saturation" Treatment Doses

These involve taking whole heads of garlic at one sitting and are usually used to purge the body of some serious or deep-seated complaint. A traditional Chinese treatment for tuberculosis involves taking 30 g (1 oz) on the first day (equivalent to ten average cloves, or about one smallish head of garlic) and working up to 90–120 g (3–4 oz) during a period of " purgation," then reducing to 30 g (1 oz) a day again for 3 months. At the same time, the patient inhales garlic fumes several times a day and has its juice in oil rubbed on his back. Russian folk medicine uses saturation doses, one head of garlic to a cup of milk, for whooping cough, dysentery, seizures, and as an enema for threadworms. Marcovici used a bulb a day to treat dysentery.

The American study on reducing high blood pressure began with a dose of 35 g (about $1\frac{1}{4}$ oz) of fresh juice, corresponding to about four heads. Few of the subjects could stomach this in one go, so a dose corresponding to two bulbs was settled on; this is the limit agreed on by most scientists as a tolerable dose for one sitting. The

Indians of the Bower manuscript, however, clearly believed that it was both safe and therapeutically useful to push the patient beyond this limit.

> . . . the fresh juice of garlic, strained through a piece of
> cloth . . . there is no fixed measure. While he is drink-
> ing, one should gently blow on him soft currents of air
> with a fan made of palm leaves; and if he swoons whilst
> drinking one should sprinkle him with cold water and
> rub him with paste of sandal.

Medium "Regular" Treatment Doses

On the basis of evidence and also of common sense, we would consider an appropriate standard medicinal dose of garlic to be around three cloves a day. You cannot expect garlic to act against infections at doses much less than this. Michael Tierra's syrup, which appears later in this chapter, is a carefully-thought-out preparation and comes from his manual *The Way of Herbs;* the dose he recommends corresponds to around nine grams or three cloves a day. The *British Herbal Pharmacopoeia,* the semi-official reference book for herbalists, calls for two to four grams of the bulb three times a day. There are other folk cures and preparations which recommend about one clove three times a day. This is not an excessive amount. We have already mentioned the Jains and the Chinese of Ganshan county who happily consume a head a day, sick or well.

The doses in scientific studies often go up to saturation levels because they are looking for decisive, short-term effects. The blood's tendency to clot is the most sensitive of all measures of garlic's action; here researchers achieved measurable reductions with a clove a day and less. However, when the doses given in scientific studies went much below what we have called regular, the effects faded.

Minimum, "Heart-Care" Preventive Doses

In this category are doses of one clove a day. This may be more acceptable to northern Europeans unused to garlic, as it is only appropriate for a very gentle, long-term treatment or as a mild preventive measure. Such a dose is effective in reducing blood clotting and choles-terol levels, when taken over a considerable period.

How to Take Fresh Garlic

There are many ways of taking garlic medicinally, but none can compare with a tooth-and-nail assault on a fresh clove. In that way you get the most allicin, so as discussed in the last chapter, fresh garlic is best for dealing with all kinds of infections—digestive troubles, bronchi-tis, abseses, and so on. The first essential operation is to crush garlic; the garlic must be thoroughly broken up so that as little as possible remains solid. The best way is to mash it in a blender into a homogenous paste. If there is insufficient bulk, add an onion but do not count it in the dosage. A meat grinder or garlic press is the second-best method. Otherwise cut the clove into as small pieces as possible, place them on a board, cover with the flat of a knife and press with your fist. Put the crushed garlic into a glass of lukewarm water and mix, adding honey to taste. As you drink it down, chew up what remains of the solids. This is important, since even a presser leaves a lot uncrushed and, if you do not pulverize it now, it will simply go through you undigested like any other vegetable fiber. Try to have water in your mouth as you chew, as this lessens the burning taste.

There are various preparations which you can make up yourself. You may find it more convenient to have one of these on hand, rather than go through the process of crushing each time. We give detailed instructions on how to make up these preparations at the end of this chapter. There may be certain advantages in taking them. We recommend using the oil for infections such as those of the ear, or where the fresh juice irritates the skin. The syrups are designed to sooth soreness of the throat and to be easy on an upset digestion. A these preparations to have been let stand. So the unstable allicin will change to diallyl disulphide and other sulphides. For "heating" the body, for the circulation, as a mild treatment for sore throat, and as an anti-toxin, these preparations are therefore perfectly effective. However, they will be less potent against bacteria and fungi than fresh garlic. If you want to make up a preparation which will be as rich in allicin as possible, then use Monsignor Greenstock's anti-infective recipe, which is designed for this purpose.

The same considerations arise when one considers whether it is better to take garlic fresh or after it has been cooked. Pliny, surprisingly perhaps, thought it more useful cooked than raw. Dioscorides thought that both cleared a cough and herbalists have argued it back and forth ever since. With the support of science, we would say that heating, like age, destroys the allicin and, again, makes it lose its anti-infective properties though retaining others. Cooked garlic is just as good for the circulation, as long as it is first cut or crushed. If it is cooked whole and untouched, neither allicin nor diallyl disulphide will be formed and it will have only minimal medicinal properties.

Many remedies call for consumption three times a day. There is good reason for this. Scientific studies on diallyl disulphide show that it is oxidized to sulphate in the liver and eliminated within three or four hours. Dr. Boullin's work on blood clotting demonstrated that garlic's effect lasted about three hours. So doses taken throughout the day will best maintain its presence in the body.

RECIPES FOR REMEDIES

Garlic for Everything

This part of the chapter gives detailed instructions on preparing and taking fresh garlic. In this first group are methods suitable for every kind of condition. This includes all kinds of internal infections, even, for example, cystitis, since garlic rapidly and easily permeates all parts of the body. External infections can also be helped by eating garlic; it is strongly recommended for some types of eczema and for acne, since it helps remove the internal impurities causing the eruptions.

Fresh Garlic
1. Chew a clove. This, if you can do it, is especially good for sinus infections, as the vapor rises upwards.
2. Chew a clove in two tablespoons of yogurt or sour cream.

3. Crush a clove and mix in lukewarm water, adding honey to taste.
4. Crush a clove and mix in warm milk.

Take one clove three times a day, with meals.

Water Extract
This is Monsignor Greenstock's extract, rich in allicin. The onion enhances the medicinal properties of the garlic.

> 50 g (1³/₄ oz) of finely chopped garlic, previously frozen
> 25 g (just under 1 oz) of finely chopped onion, previously frozen
> 200 ml (¹/₃ pt) of 23% alcohol (or if unavailable, we recommend vodka and water in equal proportions)
> 1 ml (¹/₄ teaspoon) ascorbic acid solution (or 1 g of Vitamin C)

Mix in a blender; let stand for two weeks at 4 C (39 F), i.e. in the refrigerator. Store the liquid in dark glass bottles. Add a few drops of oil of mint or cloves. It lasts up to eight months. A "regular" dose would be 1–2 teaspoons three times a day, with meals.

Garlic Pearls or Tablets: A Reminder on Dosage
For those who find them more convenient or palatable than fresh garlic, we repeat the dosages recommended in the last chapter. For a "regular" dose, take sufficient oil capsules to give you 3 mg of oil three times a day, or 9 mg in all. The oil can also be extracted from the capsule by piercing it with a pin, and used for ear infections or external application. Dried garlic in tablet or other forms has lost its water, which comprises $^2/_3$ of the weight of fresh garlic. So 1 g of dried garlic is equivalent to 3 g of

fresh garlic. For a regular treatment dose of tablets containing garlic powder, take 1 g three times a day, or 3 g ($^1/_3$ oz) in all. For a mild, preventive dose, take 1 g in total per day.

Gentler Garlic

The second group contains remedies designed to help the chest and head complaints listed in our table, or to be used in cases where fresh garlic would cause irritation.

Syrups

This is based on Michael Tierra's syrup. Put 250 g (8 oz) of minced or crushed garlic in a 1 l or 2 pt wide-mouthed jar. Almost fill with equal parts of apple-cider vinegar and distilled water. Cover and let stand in a warm place for four days, shaking a few times a day. Add 1 cup of glycerine and let stand for a day. Strain through a cloth, add 1 cup of honey, and stir thoroughly. Keep cool. For deep-seated coughs, sore throats, chronic bronchitis, high blood pressure, and circulation problems, take 1 tablespoon three times a day with meals.

A simpler syrup: Pour 0.5 l (1 pt) of boiling water over 60 g (2 oz) of minced or crushed garlic. Keep in a cool place for 10 hours. Strain, and add 1 tablespoonful of vinegar and enough honey to make a syrup. Sip 1 tablespoonful three times a day as an expectorant.

To this can be added:

a) 15 g ($^1/_2$ oz) of grated horseradish. This is a Polish practice; it encourages sweating and so is good for bronchitis.

b) 15 g ($^1/_2$ oz) bruised fennel and caraway seeds. This

encourages and soothes the stomach and so is good for digestive problems.

Sage Garlic Tea and Gargle

Brew 2 tablespoons of dried sage and four or five minced or crushed cloves of garlic in 1 l (2 pt) of boiling water. Cover and stand until lukewarm. Take 1 small teacupful four or five times a day and gargle every half hour. For tonsillitis and to reduce mucus.

An Inhalant

Take three or four cloves of minced or crushed garlic and a teaspoon of apple vinegar. Add .5 l (1 pt.) of boiling water and inhale the fumes. For nasal congestion.

External Remedies

Here are ways in which garlic can be applied externally to the skin. There are advantages in getting it as close as possible to the site of the infection, provided care is taken to keep the surrounding area free from possible blistering and provided you are prepared to put up with some initial stinging. If it burns too much, let it stand for a few minutes and try again.

Poultices

To apply garlic to a small area, first put petroleum jelly on the skin around it to prevent blistering. Put a small amount of minced garlic onto a piece of gauze and tape it in place with adhesive tape. Leave it on for 15–30 minutes. For athlete's foot, abscesses, boils, and other skin infections.

To treat and soothe a wider area, you can use this bread poultice. Finely grate 60 g (2 oz) of garlic and add a crumbled 450 g (1 lb) wheat meal loaf soaked in cold milk. Apply to the skin.

For treating acne, spots, and mouth ulcers, simply hold or rub a bruised clove against the place.(Russians used to press a half walnut shell filled with crushed garlic to the skin as a means of getting it into the system, but that was in the days before adhesive tape.)

From Russia: Mix equal parts of zinc-oxide ointment, lanolin, and ground garlic (preferably fresh garlic ground in a blender). As always, use a glass or ceramic container, not a metal one. Store in a covered jar. For eczema and hemorrhoids.

From the Anglo-Saxon *Leech Book*: Take elecampane, garlic, chervil, radish, turnip, raven's foot, honey, and pepper. Pound the plants and boil them in the honey. For a "wensalve," an ointment for boils and swellings.

Garlic in Oil

Mince or crush 250 g (8 oz) of garlic and put it in a wide jar. Add enough olive oil to cover the garlic. Close the jar tightly and shake a few times a day. Stand it in a warm place for three days, then strain through a cloth. Keep the mixture cool. For earaches, put a few drops, warmed, in the ear on some cotton wool. For aches, sprains, and minor skin disorders, rub on; heating may help to ease pain. You can also add essential oils such as eucalyptus, cypress, or myrrh to the oil.

Mix together 10 tablespoons castor oil and ten cloves of minced garlic. Cover and leave for thirty-six hours then strain and bottle. This mixture is recommended as a hair conditioner. Massage it into the hair and scalp and wrap the head in a warm towel. After an hour, shampoo the hair normally. This application is also useful for removing head lice and nits.

A Suppository
Scrape a clove to produce juice, insert it into the rectum, and leave overnight. Repeat as needed. For hemorrhoids. (Also for hemorrhoids is this Russian remedy: put a very hot brick in a pail with a hole in the lid. Put pieces of raw garlic on it to burn and sit over the fumes!)

Additional Remedies

History provides us with a wealth of garlic concoctions. Here are a few which took our fancy and also appealed to our common sense.

Four Thieves' Vinegar
This is supposedly what the thieves drank to prevent them getting the Plague (see chapter 4). It is described as antiseptic and very aromatic.

Take 7 g (¼ oz) each of calamus root, cinnamon, ground nutmeg, lavender, mint, rosemary, rue, sage and wormwood, and two minced heads of garlic. Add 1 l (2 pt) of cider vinegar. Cover and keep warm for five days. Strain and add 7 g (¼ oz) of powdered camphor before bottling.

An Anglo-Saxon Bronchial Remedy
"Flag and feverfew, garlic and radish, the inside of helenium bark, and cress, nettle, peppermint that grows

by the stream. Take malt-ale and pour it over the plants for nine nights. Give to drink fasting." This recipe is found in Cockayne's *Leechdoms, Wortcunning and Starcraft of Early England.* The same text recommends for tightness of the chest "a great deal of garlic."

A Roman Aphrodisiac
"Garlic is believed to act as an aphrodisiac, when pounded with fresh coriander and taken in neat wine." So said Gaius Pliny.

Garlic Brandy
Steep three or four crushed cloves in a small bottle of brandy in a dark cupboard for fourteen days. Such a tincture was recommended in the eighteenth century by Dr. James Lind for seamen on cold winter journeys. "A man will find a much less quantity of it than of the Pure Spirit warm his stomach; and it will keep the Breast, Skin and Kidneys free from Obstructions."

A Siberian Energy Food
Mince four heads of garlic and four fresh onions. Boil 250 g (8 oz) of barley in 0.9 l (2 pt) of water until all the liquid is gone; do the same with 250 g (8 oz) of oats, then mince both grains. Mince 60 g (2 oz) of dried valerian root. Combine all these with 1 kg (2 lb) of honey until it is like a thick cream. Spread it 2.5 cm (1 in) thick and let it set for a day. Cut it into 2.5 cm (1 in) squares. Take three to six a day.

Instant Recovery Soup
If you have been ill, there is nothing like this easy-to-

prepare soup to get you back on your feet. Put 2 full teaspoons miso, 1–2 cloves crushed garlic, a little grated onion, and a squeeze of lemon in a mug or bowl. Add boiling water or vegetable stock, and mix well. Add a dash of soy sauce to taste.

Garlic to Heal the Garden

Do not forget that garlic will help protect your plants as well as yourself (and your pets). Here again is Monsignor Greenstock's home insecticide, and something to keep the insects off us human beings as well.

An Insecticide
Soak thirty minced cloves of garlic in 2 teaspoons (10 ml) mineral oil (e.g. paraffin) for twenty-four hours. Dissolve 7 g (¼ oz) of an oil-based soap in 600 ml (1 pt) of water and add it to the garlic, stirring thoroughly. Strain and store the liquid in a glass or ceramic container. Use it as a spray on your plants at a dilution of between 1 part in 20 and 1 part in 100 of water.

An Insect Repellent
Take 1 cup of sunflower or sesame seed oil, ½ cup of fresh feverfew (*Tanacetum parthenium*) or tansy *(Tanacetum vulgare)* flowers, or 1 tablespoon of the dried flowers, and eight cloves of minced garlic. Simmer the oil and blossoms for 15 minutes, cool and add the garlic. Bottle the mixture and keep it for five days, shaking two or three times a day, then strain. It can also be used as a remedy for bites.

Garlic Cookery

Cooking with garlic is a subject of its own and we have not attempted to go into it in this book. It is certainly coming into its own in the United States, and there are even one or two cookbooks devoted entirely to garlic recipes. We recommend taking garlic in your diet, so here are some basic recipes to start with. If you can get organically grown food as well as garlic, you will find a taste as well as health advantage.

Garlic Butter

Crush two or three cloves of garlic and mix into 120 g (4 oz) of melted butter. Stir over a low heat for a few minutes and add a small bunch of parsley, finely chopped. Continue to stir until the parsley has wilted. Put the butter into a container to set. If you are worried about the cholesterol in the butter, remember that the garlic will reduce it.

Garlic Bread

Crush two or three cloves of garlic, add a little salt and stir into 120 g (4 oz) of melted butter. Slice a French loaf lengthwise and spread both sides with the butter. Place the two halves together again and wrap in foil. Bake for 10 minutes at 200 C (400 F).

Garlic Spaghetti

Put spaghetti in boiling salted water. When spaghetti is half cooked, add three or four cloves of sliced, fried garlic, and 4 tablespoons olive oil, with pepper and salt.

Finish cooking spaghetti. Drain and cover with grated cheese.

Garlic Broth

Take just over 1 l (2½ pt) of vegetable broth or stock. Add six chopped cloves of garlic, 1½ tablespoons of olive oil, and half a bay leaf. Add rice or noodles if required. Simmer for 20 minutes. Just before it is done, add ¼ teaspoon thyme and a pinch of sage.

So, having prepared your garlic, be prepared for anything. It will give you health, energy, and a zest for life, and you do not know down what paths it may lead you.

12

Garlic Prospect

Today there are more doubts about the wisdom and effectiveness of modern scientific medicine than at any time since its origins. Those who attack it use much the same argument as did the Galenicists and herbal doctors whom it replaced—that it ignores the patient as a whole person, to his peril, and is only concerned with his disease. Only now are the full consequences of this being realized. Two out of five people who receive a drug in the hospital suffer from drug side effects. Half of all adults take a drug of some kind every day. Major overall improvements could be made through prevention, through encouraging better diet and healthier life-styles, but very little effort is made in these directions. In the major industrial countries, around 0.5% of health care expenditure goes toward prevention and, instead, resources are put into expensive, last-minute measures such as heart and kidney transplants, hip replacements, and other radical surgery.

Large numbers of people are turning back to modern

medicine's historical rivals such as acupuncture and natural remedies. More than half of the United States population is eating healthier food and taking food supplements.
Twenty million people in the United States pay an annual visit to a chiropractor.

Herbs and herbalism have been at the center of this
revival. Their pervasive, preventive, and generally harmless action is in sharp contrast to the powerful, specific,
and often toxic effects of conventional drugs. The home
medicine chest may soon be as likely to contain mint or
camomile to relax an upset stomach, valerian for sleepless
nights, passiflora for stress and anxiety, salix (willow) against
pain and headaches, and comfrey or aloe for cuts and
scratches, as paracetamol, antacids, tranquilizers, or antiseptic ointments. However, there is still considerable
confusion about the real value of herbs compared with
conventional treatments or no treatment at all. How
powerful are herbs and how useful? In this chapter, we
shall address these questions with reference to garlic.

Garlic, we should remember, built its reputation when
herbs were the only medicines and their effectiveness
was a matter of life and death. Because of the generally
unsanitary living conditions, a cut could lead to gan-
grene—every doctor had seen a colleague die of a
pinprick—and diseases like tuberculosis were widespread
and lethal. Improvements in nutrition, hygiene, and sani-
tation during the latter part of the nineteenth century
led to great reductions in disease. At much the same
time, chemists were synthesizing new, chemically-pure
drugs which, in certain cases, had dramatically successful
effects; a little aspirin brought down a fever in twenty
minutes and the drug salvarsan, produced at the turn of

the century, cured the hitherto incurable syphilis. These two kinds of advance, in hygiene and in drugs, were linked together in people's minds as products of reason and science.

As a result, herbs were thought of as part of the ignorant, unscientific past and went out of fashion—there are fashions in medicine as in almost every other aspect of life. The new medicines could be dispensed in exact dosages and directed against specific diseases; herbs were annoyingly vague in their effects and their strengths varied from dose to dose. Gradually they were removed from the pharmacopeia, the official lists of drugs. This was not because they were ineffective—there was never any proper assessment of their effectiveness—but they simply did not fit the new medical outlook. The chemically pure drugs forged ahead. In the 1930s there were the sulpha drugs, from the 1940s on there was penicillin and other antibiotics and, in many cases, these could save lives in a spectacular way. They could certainly treat acute and dangerous diseases more reliably than many herbs. But now we know that modern drugs are strong and relatively toxic and should only be used where absolutely necessary. Health-conscious people have been forced to think again about these drugs and not take them unless there is no choice. All too often short-term comfort and fast recovery have been bought at the cost of long-term health. Some antibiotic and antifungal agents, for example, can reduce vitality, disturb the digestion, produce allergies, or cause candida infections. At the same time they may make the body more vulnerable to the disease and increase the chances of infection returning at a later date, as urethritis or cystitis sufferers know. For this reason antibiotics shouldn't be taken for every sore throat or minor infection, but taken, of course, for pneumonia. It is much better to control blood pressure and cholesterol levels with diet. But if your blood pressure suddenly jumps way up, or drops way down—don't hesitate to go to a doctor.

The variety of effects of an herb may be a great asset, not a disadvantage, because the herbal remedy treats ill health in several different ways. For example, if you take garlic for a nagging bronchitis, it holds back the bacteria. It also "heats" your body; you may sweat, and this helps you throw off the disease. (In traditional practice, increased urination would also be regarded as beneficial.) Metabolism is improved and poisons are removed. All this happens without cost to your vitality. And also, of course, without cost to your pocket. In most cases, this treatment will be effective if combined with other measures, such as a diet free from milk products and refined foods; other herbs, like coltsfoot and sage, which help the cough and dry up secretions, can also be used. By comparison, modern treatments for chronic bronchitis are minimal. There are expectorants which are supposed to help you cough up the phlegm, but which are known to be relatively useless. There are cough suppressants, like codeine, which may drive the infection deeper. Antibiotics are given only if the infection suddenly becomes acute. Clearly you have nothing much to lose by trying garlic for bronchitis. Likewise, garlic's multiple effects on the circulation—reducing cholesterol and fat production and blood clotting, and moderating high blood pressure—could only be matched by a combination of conventional drugs, which would have a series of interacting side effects.

Herbs have another advantage: they can both prevent

and cure, using the same principles. Garlic reduces the cholesterol content of a fatty meat meal long before any abnormalities appear in the circulation. When you travel abroad, taking garlic in normal doses helps you cope with unfamiliar bacteria and prevents an upset stomach; this is surely what Pliny and many other herbalists meant by it being "of great benefit against changes of water and residence." In larger doses, it will treat stomach infections. Modern antibiotics, on the other hand, cannot be used preventively; you cannot take penicillin all the time. When this is tried, as in the constant dosing of intensively farmed hens or calves, the animals become breeding grounds for stronger and more resistant organisms; the connection between this and a considerable recent increase in cases of salmonella and food poisoning is now being admitted.

This question of resistance is an important one. So far as anyone knows, no organisms have ever become resistant to garlic. There is not enough experience to show that it could never happen. However, garlic's effects on cells are probably so wide ranging, that a cell which altered sufficiently to avoid them would alter itself out of existence.

Herbs in general, and garlic in particular, do have certain disadvantages, though these can be surmounted. One is that not all preparations are of the same strength—the chemists had a valid point. The way a bulb is grown, extracted, concentrated, stored, and prepared for consumption will alter its potency. The problem existed in earlier days, but at least there were guides to preparation and doses in the official pharmacopeia. Entries on herbs remained there until well into this century, but now there are no official standards and no control in the market place. We can solve this problem by consumer power. Consumers should, if possible, only buy herb products which have the amount of active ingredients written on the packet. This would encourage manufacturers to carry out lab tests for minimum levels of active ingredients, as well as purity and quality. In the case of garlic, buy products that have a statement about allicin levels as well as actual garlic content on the packet.

The second disadvantage is that garlic, like other herbs, is not an exactly-targeted weapon. It may not always work, or its effect may sometimes be too weak. The professional therapist who uses herbs is trained to expect this and he will know how to adopt a strategic approach involving a combination of herbs and methods. A professional therapist should be consulted for proper treatment for persistent infections, serious stomach problems, or cardiovascular disease. He should tackle your condition at its source and should also decide if garlic is or is not the right remedy in your particular case. As far as home use is concerned, the best insurance against failure is knowledge and experience; you should learn how you respond in different circumstances, what are the best preparations for you and the right times to use them. Consider, for example, which kinds of health problems you are likely to get, and research the herbs which can prevent and treat these problems. Which times are you more likely to pick up infections: at the onset of winter, perhaps? At the same time garlic should not be looked upon as infallible or asked to do things it cannot do. If you are seriously ill, you must seek professional help immediately.

It is our view that modern drugs are an advance in

medical knowledge, that they have saved many lives and that it would be pure foolishness to abandon them completely in favor of herbs. However, we also feel they are used too much. First should come natural preventive measures, herbs among them; modern drugs should be a standby when all else has failed. Then one would get the best of both worlds or, as the Chinese aim for in their national medicine, "the best of the old and the new."

Of course, garlic itself might well become the basis for new chemically pure drugs. At present, one cannot patent the products of nature, so a company which researches and develops a plant acquires no exclusive rights. Pharmaceutical companies therefore have strong motives for converting natural substances into patentable chemicals. We guess that a new garlic-based anti-clotting chemical drug is being quietly tested somewhere. If such a thing does appear, it may not have any particular advantages over a proper use of the natural bulb and it will certainly be more expensive. Garlic, like all other plants, has an enormous number of constituents; some of them are known, and some of their effects are understood, but there is always more to know and understand. Allicin, diallyl disulphide, MATS and DITS, and ajoene are medically effective, but who knows what other constituents have unexpected powers or help to make the whole mixture healthy and harmless to man?

Garlic has so ancient a reputation and is so safe that national regulatory bodies the world over accept preparations of it. In the United States, they are classed as foods and were on the *Generally Recognized as Safe* (GRAS) list. In Britain, the sale of garlic products is not restricted in any way. The law in Britain is more relaxed, and manufacturers of garlic products there are allowed to claim:

> A herbal remedy traditionally used for the treatment of the symptoms of the common cold and cough. A herbal remedy traditionally used for the temporary relief of symptoms of rhinitis and catarrh.

In Germany the government-appointed "Commission E" has defined garlic's effectiveness, and allowed claims that it can be used together with diet to bring down blood cholesterol, and that it can help prevent atherosclerosis.

There remains the problem of garlic's smell, which still discourages many people. Things are changing, but its complete social acceptance is still far in the future. Much of the reaction against it is just cultural conditioning, the kind of prejudice which led people to eat white bread and white sugar because it was more sophisticated and to prefer medicines in the form of sterilized white pills. Today, however, organic is sophisticated, and the more we realize the benefits of eating fresh garlic, the more we will come to like and accept it. Natural remedies have natural smells. Let us give the last word on the matter to Sir John Harington, writing in 1607:

> *Sith Garlicke then hath power to save from death,*
> *Bear with it though it make unsavory breath,*
> *And scorne not Garlicke, like some that thinke*
> *It only makes men winke, and drinke, and stinke.*

Recommended Reading

A Note on Sources

The material of the first four chapters has been gathered from a great number of sources, far too numerous to list in full. The authors and their books are often mentioned directly in the text and interested readers may consult them, in translation where necessary, looking in indexes and tables of contents under garlic, garleke, allium and so on. Pliny's account of the medicinal properties, for example, is to be found in Book 20, Chapter 23, of his *Natural History*. The quotations from Hippocrates come from the complete French translations of his canon. An account of the varieties of *Allium* and of the botanical origins of garlic are to be found in the 1944 issue of the periodical *Herbertia*. The Bower manuscript was edited and translated by Rudolf Hoernle and published in 1893; we have had its list retranslated. The only full English translation of Dioscorides' *Materia Medica* was made in 1655. L.J. Harris, in his *Book on Garlic*, gives a more modern translation of the passage on garlic and refers to the German version of J. Berendes. Harris has far and away the most amusing collection of material on garlic and also a useful bibliography. However, much of what he says is taken from secondary sources. It is always wise to check originals; for example, Herodotus' visit to the Great Pyramid is described in his *History,* Book Two, Chapter 75, and says nothing about the workers going on strike when they did not get their usual rations of garlic. Nor does Aristophanes say anything about garlic and Olympic athletes.

The scientific papers consulted are also too numerous to be listed in full. We have made a selection of the most important ones, arranged in alphabetical order by subject. We are fortunate in having two comprehensive scientific monographs on garlic published within the last few years. There is the review by Fenwick and Hanley, and the book by Koch and Hahn, published in German. The latter quotes approximately 1000 references on garlic.

References

Books and Articles on Garlic

Fenwick, G.G. and Hanley, A.B. (1984). The Genus Allium. *CRC Critical Reviews in Food Science and Nutrition 22:* 199–377; *23:* 1–73.

Fulder, S. (1989). *Garlic: Lifeblood of Good Health.* Thorsons: Wellingborough, U.K.

Greenstock, D. (1976). Las propriades terapeuticas del ajo. *Ceres* Oct/Nov/Dec.

Harris, L. (1979). *The Book of Garlic.* Panjandrum/Aris, Los Angeles.

Koch, H.P. and Hahn, G. (1988). *Knoblauch.* Urban & Schwarzenberg: Munich, Baltimore.

Leclerc, H. (1918). Histoire de l'ail. *Janus 23:* 167–91

Watanabe, T. (1974). *Garlic Therapy*. Japan Publications: San Francisco.

Garlic Cookery

Gilroy Garlic Festival Association (1980). *The Garlic Lover's Cookbook*. Celestial Arts: Berkeley, California.

Shulman, M.R. (1984). *Garlic Cookery*. Thorsons: Wellingborough, U.K.

General Background

Fulder, S. (1988). *The Handbook of Complementary Medicine*. Oxford University Press: Oxford; New York.

Grieve, M. (1976). *A Modern Herbal*. Penguin Books: Middlesex, U.K.; New York.

Kourenoff, P. and St. George, G. (1970). *Russian Folk Medicine*. W.H. Allen: New York.

Lewis, W.H. and Lewis, M.P.F.(1977). *Medical Botany*. Wiley: New York.

Tierra, M. (1980). *The Way of Herbs*. Washington Square Pocket Books, Simon & Schuster: New York.

Chemistry

Block, E. (1985). The Chemistry of Garlic and Onions. *Sci. Am.* 252 (3): 94–7

Brodnitz, M.H., et al. (1971). Flavour Components of Garlic Extract *J. Agric. Food Chem.* 19: 273–5

Cavallito, L.C., et al. (1944). Allicin, the Antibacterial Principle of *Allium sativum*. 1. Isolation, Physical Properties and Antibacterial Action. *J. Am. Chem. Soc.* 66: 1950, 1952–4.

Iberl, B., et al. (1990). Quantitative Determination of Allicin and Alliin from Garlic by HPLC. *Planta Medica* 56: 320–326.

Jansen, H., Mueller, B., and Knobloch, K. (1987). Allicin Characterisation and Its Determination by HPLC. *Planta Medica* 53: 559–562.

Lawson, L.D. and Hughes, B.G. (1989) Analysis of Aqueous Garlic Extract & Garlic Products by HPLC. *Planta Medica 55:* 639.

Stoll, A. and Seebeck, E. (1951). Chemical Investigations on Alliin, the Specific Principle of Garlic. *Adv. Enzymol. 11:* 377–400.

Infections

Adetumbi, M.A. and Lau, B.H.S. (1983). Allium sativum (Garlic) — a Natural Antibiotic. *Med. Hypotheses 12:* 227–37.

Caporaso, N., Smith, S.M., and Eng. R.H.F (1983). Antifungal Activity in Human Urine and Serum after Ingestion of Garlic (Allium sativum). *Antimicrob. Agents Chemother. 23:* 700–702.

Damrau, F. and Ferguson, E.A. (1949). The Therapeutic Value of Garlic in Functional Gastrointestinal Disorders. *Rev. Gastroenterol. 16:* 411–19.

Ghannoum, M.A. (1988). Studies on the Anticandidal mode of action of Allium sativum (garlic). *J. Gen Microb. 134:* 2917–2924.

Hitokoto, M., et al. (1978). Inhibitory effects of condiments and herbal drugs on the growth and toxin production of toxigenic fungi. *Mycopathologia 66:* 161–7.

Johnson, M.J. and Vaughan, R.H. (1969). Death of *Salmonella typhimurium* and *Escherichia coli* in the presence of freshly re-constituted dehydrated garlic and onion. *Appl. Microbiol. 17:* 903–905.

Kumar, A. and Sharma, V.D. (1982). Inhibitory effect of garlic on enterotoxigenic *Escherichia coli. Ind. J. Med. Res. 76:* 66–70.

Mirelman, D., et al. (1987). Inhibition of growth of entamoeba histolytica by allicin, the active principle of garlic extract (Allium sativum). *J. Infections Dis. 156:* 243–244.

Moore, G.S. and Atkins (1977). The fungicidal and fungistatic activity of an aqueous garlic extract on medically important yeast-like fungi. *Mycologia, 69:* 341–348.

Sandhu, D.K., et al. (1980). Sensitivity of yeasts isolated from cases of vaginitis to aqueous extracts of garlic. *Mykosen 23:* 691–98.

Sharma, V.D., et al. (1977). Antibacterial property of Allium sativum: in vivo and in vitro studies. *Ind. J. Exp. Biol. 15:* 466–8.

Tsai, Y., et al. (1985). Antiviral properties of garlic: in vitro effects on Influenza B, Herpes simplex and Coxsackie viruses. *Planta Medica 51:* 460—1.

Blood Circulation, Cholesterol, Fats, and Coagulation

Arora, R.C. and Arora, S. (1981). Comparative effects of clofibrate, garlic and onion on alimentary hyperlipaemia. *Atherosclerosis 39:* 447–52

Barrie, S., Wright, J., and Pizzorno, J. (1987). Effect of garlic oil on platelet aggregation, serum lipids and blood pressure in humans. *J. Orthomolecular Medicine 2:* 15–21.

Bordia, A. (1978). Effect of garlic on human platelet aggregation in vitro. *Atherosclerosis 30:* 355–60.

Bordia, A. (1981). Effect of garlic on blood lipids in patients with coronary heart disease. *Am. J. Clin. Nutr. 34:* 2100–03.

Boullin, D.J. (1981). Garlic as platelet inhibitor. *Lancet I:* 776–7.

Ernst, E., Weihmayr, T., and Matrai, A. (1985). Garlic and blood lipids. *Brit. Med. J. 291:* 391.

Grunwald, J. (1990). Garlic and Cardiovascular Risk Factors. *Brit. J. Clinical Pharmacol. 29:* 582.

Harenberg, J., Giese, C., and Zimmerman, R. (1988). Effect of dried garlic on blood co-agulation, fibrinolysis, platelet aggregation and serum cholesterol levels in patients with hyperlipoproteinemia. *Atherosclerosis 74:* 247–249.

Kendler, B.S. (1987). Garlic (Allium sativum) and onion (Allium cepa) — a review of their relationship to cardiovascular disease. *Preventive Med. 16:* 670–685.

Keys, A. (1980). Wine, garlic and coronary heart disease in seven countries. *Lancet I:* 145–6.

Kiesewetter, H., et al. (1990). Effects of garlic on blood fluidity and fibrinolytic activity: a randomised placebo — controlled double-blind study. *Brit. J. Clinical Practice,* Supplement *69:* 24–29.

Kleijnen, J., et al. (1989). Garlic, onions and cardiovascular risk factors. A review of the evidence from human experiments with emphasis on commercially available preparations. *Brit. J. Clinical Practice 28:* 535–544.

Mader, F.H. (1990). Treatment of hyperlipidaemia with garlic powder tablets. *Drug Research 40:* 3–8.

Makheja, A.N., et al. (1979). Inhibition of platelet aggregation and thromboxane synthesis by onion and garlic. *Lancet I:* 781.

Sainani, G.S., et al. (1979). Effect of dietary garlic and onion on serum lipid profile in Jain community. *Ind. J. Med. Res. 69:* 776–80.

Sainani, G.S., et al. (1976). Onion, garlic and atherosclerosis. *Lancet I:* 575–6.

Saxena, K.K., et al. (1979). Garlic in stress-induced myocardial damage. *Ind. Heart J. 31:* 187–8.

Blood Sugar and Diabetes

Chang, M.L.W. and Johnson, M.A. (1980). Effect of garlic on carbohydrate metabolism and lipid synthesis in rats. *J. Nutr. 110:* 931–36.

Matthew, P.T. and Augusti, K.T. (1973). Studies on the effect of allicin on alloxan diabetes. *Ind. J. Biochem. Biophys. 10:* (3) 209–15.

Side Effects

Nakagawa, S. (1980). Effect of raw and extracted-aged garlic juice on growth of young rats and their organs after peroral administration. *Toxicol. Sci. 5:* 91–112.

Ruffin, J. and Hunter, S.A. (1983). An evaluation of the side effects of garlic as an antihypertensive agent. *Cytobios 37:* 85–9.

Cancer and Detoxification

Belman, S. (1983). Onion and garlic oils and tumour promotion. *Carcinogensis 4:* 1063–5.

Fujiwara, M. and Natata, T. (1967). Induction of tumour immunity with tumour cells treated with extract of garlic. *Nature 216:* 83–4.

Lau, B.H. (1989). Detoxifying, radioprotective and phagocyte-enhancing effects of garlic. *Int. Clin. Nutrit. Rev. 9:* 27–31.

Nishino, et al. (1989). Antitumour-promoting activity of garlic extract. *Oncology 46:* 277–280.

Wargovich, M.J. (1987). Diallyl sulphide, a flavour component of garlic (Allium sativum) inhibits dimethylhydrazine induced colon cancer. *Carcinogenesis 8:* 487–489.

Weisberger, A.S. and Pensky, J. (1957). Tumour inhibiting effects derived from an active principle of garlic (Allium sativum). *Science 126:* 1112.

Pesticide

Amonkar, S.V. and Reeves, E.L. (1970). Mosquito control with active principle of garlic. J. *Econ. Entomol. 63:* 1172–5.

Amonkar, S.V. and Vijayalakshmi, L. (1979). Control of anthracnose disease of grape vines by garlic oil. *Trans. Br. Mycol. Soc. 73:* 350–1.

Ark, P.A. and Thompson, J.P. (1959). Control of certain diseases of plants with antibiotics from garlic. *Plant Dis. Rep. 43:* 276–82.

Index